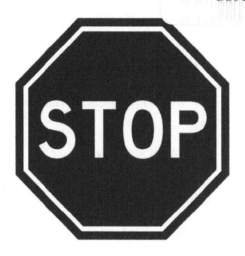

FREE Test Taking Tips DVD Offer

To help us better serve you, we have developed a Test Taking Tips DVD that we would like to give you for FREE. **This DVD covers world-class test taking tips that you can use to be even more successful when you are taking your test.**

All that we ask is that you email us your feedback about your study guide. Please let us know what you thought about it – whether that is good, bad or indifferent.

To get your **FREE Test Taking Tips DVD**, email freedvd@studyguideteam.com with "FREE DVD" in the subject line and the following information in the body of the email:

> a. The title of your study guide.

> b. Your product rating on a scale of 1-5, with 5 being the highest rating.

> c. Your feedback about the study guide. What did you think of it?

> d. Your full name and shipping address to send your free DVD.

If you have any questions or concerns, please don't hesitate to contact us at freedvd@studyguideteam.com.

Thanks again!

ATI TEAS
Study Guide
2019 & 2020

TEAS 6 Study Manual &
Practice Test Questions for the
Test of Essential Academic Skills
6th Edition

Test Prep Books

Table of Contents

Quick Overview

As you draw closer to taking your exam, effective preparation becomes more and more important. Thankfully, you have this study guide to help you get ready.

A large part of the guide is devoted to showing you what content to expect on the exam and to helping you better understand that content. Near the end of this guide is a practice test so that you can see how well you have grasped the content. Then, answer explanations are provided so that you can understand why you missed certain questions.

Once the exam is complete, take some time to relax. Even if you feel that you need to take the exam again, you will be well served by some down time before you begin studying again. It's often easier to convince yourself to study if you know that it will come with a reward!

Test-Taking Strategies

1. Predicting the Answer

When you feel confident in your preparation for a multiple-choice test, try predicting the answer before reading the answer choices. This is especially useful on questions that test objective factual knowledge or that ask you to fill in a blank. By predicting the answer before reading the available choices, you eliminate the possibility that you will be distracted or led astray by an incorrect answer choice.

2. Reading the Whole Question

Too often, test takers scan a multiple-choice question, recognize a few familiar words, and immediately jump to the answer choices. Test authors are aware of this common impatience, and they will sometimes prey upon it.

3. Looking for Wrong Answers

Long and complicated multiple-choice questions can be intimidating. One way to simplify a difficult multiple-choice question is to eliminate all of the answer choices that are clearly wrong. In most sets of answers, there will be at least one selection that can be dismissed right away.

4. Don't Overanalyze

Anxious test takers often overanalyze questions. When you are nervous, your brain will often run wild, causing you to make associations and discover clues that don't actually exist. If you feel that this may be a problem for you, do whatever you can to slow down during the test.

5. Your First Instinct

Many people struggle with multiple-choice tests because they overthink the questions. If you have studied sufficiently for the test, you should be prepared to trust your first instinct once you have carefully and completely read the question and all of the answer choices.

6. Subtle Negatives

One of the oldest tricks in the multiple-choice test writer's book is to subtly reverse the meaning of a question with a word like *not* or *except*. If you are not paying attention to each word in the question, you can easily be led astray by this trick.

Introduction

Background of the ATI TEAS

The Test of Essential Academic Skills (TEAS) is a standardized test created and distributed by Assessment Technologies Institute (ATI) to examine the test taker's aptitude for skill sets fundamental to a career in nursing. As such, the TEAS is used by nursing schools and allied health schools in the United States and Canada as a chief criterion for admission. The TEAS is currently in its sixth iteration, known as the ATI TEAS.

Test Administration

The ATI TEAS may be administered by a nursing or allied health school or a PSI testing center. Test takers can register at atitesting.com or directly through the school to which they wish to apply, as most nursing schools offer the test on-campus periodically throughout the year.

Students may retake the ATI TEAS, but most schools have limitations such as the number of days students must wait between attempts, or the number of attempts students may make in a given period.

Test Format

The ATI TEAS is comprised of 170 multiple choice questions with four possible answer choices given for each question. The questions are divided between four subject areas—Reading, Mathematics, Science, and English and Language Usage.

Subject Area	Questions	Time Limit (minutes)
Reading	53	64
Mathematics	36	54
Science	53	63
English & Language Usage	28	28
Total	**170**	**209**

Scoring

Shortly after the examination, test takers will receive several different numbered scores with their ATI TEAS results. Schools typically look at the Composite Individual Total Score.

Reading

Key Ideas and Details

Summarizing a Complex Text

A **summary** is a short paragraph of one to two sentences that describes an entire text. Summaries describe the text in the writer's own words, leaving out specific details to focus on the overall picture of the text. A simple way to write a summary is to make an outline of a complex text, then create a short paragraph describing that outline.

Example
Read the following paragraph and then answer the question.

According to the U.S. Department of Health and Human Services, 16 million people in the United States presently suffer from a smoking-related condition and nearly nine million suffer from a serious smoking-related illness. According to the Centers for Disease Control and Prevention (CDC), tobacco products cause nearly six million deaths per year. This number is projected to rise to over eight million deaths by 2030. Smokers, on average, die ten years earlier than their nonsmoking peers.

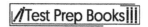

Q. Which of the following statements most accurately summarizes the paragraph?

    a. Tobacco is less healthy than many alternatives.

    b. Tobacco is deadly, and smokers would be much better off kicking the addiction.

    c. In the United States, local, state, and federal governments typically tax tobacco products, which leads to high prices.

    d. Tobacco products shorten smokers' lives by ten years and kill more than six million people per year.

Explanation

Answer. B: The author cites disease and deaths associated with smoking. Choice *B* is the correct answer because it summarizes all the details offered against smoking tobacco.

Inferring the Logical Conclusion

To **infer a logical conclusion** from a text, readers should actively read the text by making predictions, analyzing facts, and determining key words. From these clues, readers should be able to draw a logical conclusion from the text.

Example

Q. When students use inference, what are they able to do?

    a. Make logical assumptions based on contextual clues

    b. Independently navigate various types of text

    c. Summarize a text's main idea

    d. Paraphrase a text's main idea

Explanation

7. A: When a person infers something, he or she is demonstrating the ability to extract key information and make logical assumptions based on that information.

Following a Set of Directions

When presented with a set of directions, readers should start at the very beginning and read the list through carefully. If the list requests students to read everything carefully before doing anything, make sure you indeed read to the end before taking any action.

Example

The next question is based on the following directions.

Follow these instructions in chronological order to transform the word into something new.

> 1. Start with the word LOATHING.
> 2. Eliminate the first and last letter in the starting word.
> 3. Eliminate all the vowels, except I, from the word.
> 4. Eliminate the letter H from the word.

Q. What new word has been spelled?
   a. TON
   b. THIN
   c. TIN
   d. TAN

Explanation

Answer. C: After removing the first and last letter, *OATHIN* remains. Next, we eliminate all the vowels, except *I*, to get *THIN*. Finally, we remove the *H* to get *TIN*; thus, Choice *C* is the correct answer.

Specific Information from Printed Communication

The following list is an explanation of printed communication one might see in daily life.

Memo: **Memos** include a heading and a body. Within the body of the message, the information should be short and to the point.

Posted announcement: **Announcements** are found in public places and convey information in an informal way. Examples of posted announcements are items for sale, missing pets, requests for work, or business openings.

Classified ads: **Classified ads** are found in newspapers or online websites such as eBay or Craigslist. Ads are used when buying or selling items or requesting services.

Line Graphs

Line graphs are used to track changes in information over time. They have a horizontal X axis and a vertical Y axis. Dots are plotted where the X and Y axes intersect, and the dots are connected into lines. Multiple lines can also be present in a line graph to demonstrate a cluster of subjects. Let's look at an example of a simple line graph.

Example

Use the line graph to answer the following question.

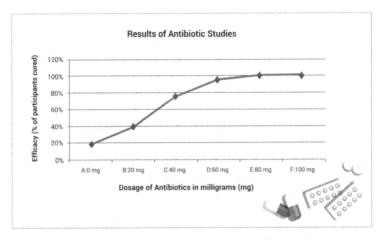

Q. What percentage of participants cured corresponds with the dosage of 20 mg?

    a. 20%

    b. 40%

    c. 60%

    d. 79%

Explanation

Answer. B: The line graph shows that at 20mg, 40% of patients were cured. The other answer choices are incorrect.

Bar Graphs

Bar graphs are useful for making comparisons between multiple variables. The multiple variables are shown on a horizontal X axis, and the bars themselves rise up on a vertical Y axis. Let's look at an example of a bar graph below.

Example
The question is based on the following bar graph.

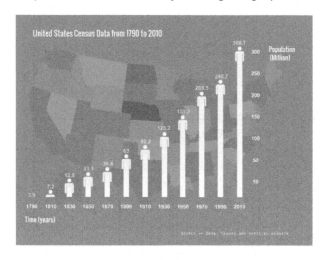

Q. In which of the following years was the United States population less than it was in 1930?

    a. 1950

    b. 1970

    c. 1910

    d. 1990

Explanation

Answer. C: The correct answer choice is C, *1910.* There are two ways to arrive at the correct answer. You could find the four answer choices on the graph, or you could have identified that the population never dips at any point. Thus, the correct answer needs to be the only answer choice that is earlier in time than the others, Choice *C.*

Pie Chart

A pie chart shows how different categories add up to 100 percent. Each category represents a "slice of the pie," and the round pie chart visually exhibits which slices are bigger or smaller than the others. Pie charts are useful for topics such as tracking finances. If the budget is represented as a pie, each chunk of the pie represents what category the finances are going to.

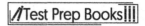

Example

The following question is based on the pie chart.

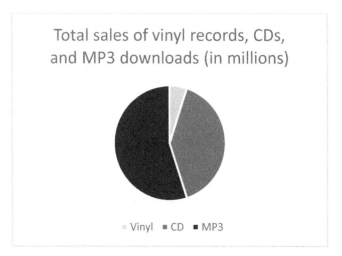

Total sales of vinyl records, CDs, and MP3 downloads (in millions)

Vinyl CD MP3

Q. This chart indicates how many sales of CDs, vinyl records, and MP3 downloads occurred over the last year. Approximately what percentage of the total sales was from CDs?

    a. 55%

    b. 25%

    c. 40%

    d. 5%

Explanation

Answer. C: The sum total percentage of a pie chart must equal 100%. Since the CD sales take up less than half of the chart and more than a quarter (25%), it can be determined to be 40% overall. This can also be measured with a protractor. The angle of a circle is 360°. Since 25% of 360 would be 90° and 50% would be 180°, the angle percentage of CD sales falls in between.

Scale Readings

Being able to read scales is important; most scales today are digitized, but there are some that still use the traditional scaled reading, such as rulers or some doctor's scales. On rulers, one side represents inches, and the other side represents centimeters. The long black lines on the inches side indicates the inch mark, with half lines between them that indicates a half-inch.

Example

Examine the three rulers below and the line being measured.

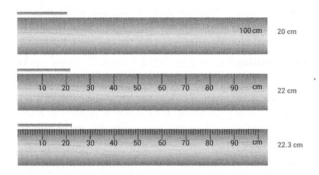

Explanation

While the length of the line remains the same, the different calibrations of the rulers result in answers with a different number of significant figures. The top ruler cannot even give a level of certainty to the ones place, so the appropriate number of significant figures is 1. The middle ruler does have a calibration that allows a measurement to the ones place so there are two significant figures. The bottom ruler can record a reading with 3 significant figures.

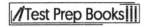

Legends and Map Keys

Legends and map keys are symbols or colors on a map that represent public parks, national or state highways, railroads, or other important landmarks. These symbols can usually be found on the bottom right corner of a map. Scales on maps may also be useful; these show relative distances between fixed points.

Example

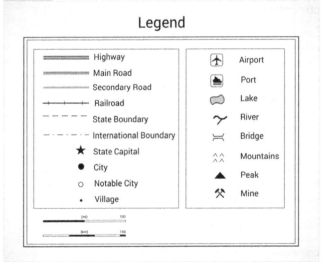

Evaluating Product Information to Determine the most Economical Buy

With the most economical buy, customers should check the fine print on the label and see the price per unit, square foot, or ounce. This will allow customers to determine the best price based on the amount. Let's look at one more example.

Example
Let's say a customer goes into a grocery store looking to buy paper towels. One brand of paper towels has five rolls for $5.86. Another brand of paper towels also has five rolls, but for $7.80. Looking for the most economical buy, the customer realizes that, although the first brand is less money, the second brand has twice as much towel on the roll. The first brand is $0.05 per square foot, while the second brand is $0.03 per square foot.

Explanation
Although the second brand costs more, it is the most economical buy, so the customer chooses the second brand.

Recognizing Events in a Sequence

The sequence of events in a story is the timeline of how the story happens. This is also known as the **plot**.

Typically, a story will go through the following plot elements: exposition, rising action, climax, falling action, and resolution. The **exposition** is the beginning of the story and usually introduces setting, characters, and conflict. In the **rising action**, readers get to know the characters better, and the **conflict** builds and builds until it reaches the climax. The **climax** is the height of the conflict. The **falling action** is when tension decreases from the conflict. Finally, the **resolution** offers solutions or an ending to the story.

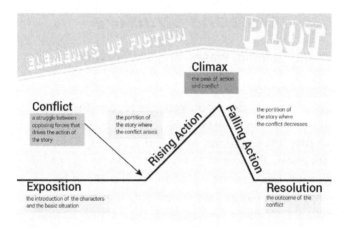

ELEMENTS OF FICTION

PLOT

Climax
the peak of action and conflict

Conflict
a struggle between opposing forces that drives the action of the story

the portition of the story where the conflict arises

Rising Action

Falling Action

the portition of the story where the conflict decreases

Exposition
the introduction of the characters and the basic situation

Resolution
the outcome of the conflict

Example

Q. Which best describes the **plot** in fiction?

a. What happens in the story or the storyline
b. Character development
c. The time and place of the story
d. The events in the story that are true

Explanation

Answer. A: The plot describes what happens in the storyline, or the sequence of events.

Craft and Structure

Fact and Opinion, Biases, and Stereotypes

Fact and Opinion

Information that can be proven true is considered factual. **Facts** can be proven by scientific experiments, mathematical equations, or by corroborating information. If I say $2 + 2 = 5$, this information can be disproven, because the equation $2 + 2 = 4$ can be proven true. **Opinions** are statements that are debatable. Opinions are not facts; that is, they cannot be proven or disproven. Examples of opinions are subjective topics such as morals, rights, and values. One person might value honesty more than kindness, but another person might value kindness higher than honesty. Neither is correct, but a matter of opinion.

Biases and Stereotypes

A **bias** is an individual prejudice that ignores evidence contrary to the belief. To prefer people who wear green hats to people who wear purple hats is to hold a favorable bias toward people who wear green hats. Biases ca be favorable or unfavorable. A **stereotype** is a widely-held belief projected onto an entire group. Those who make stereotypes fail to consider individuals within the group and how they might differentiate from that group. Stereotypes and biases can be harmful toward the groups they target; it is important for those who hold biases and stereotypes to be self-aware of those judgments and understand the harm stereotypes can have when directed toward a specific group of people.

Example

Q. Which of the following is an opinion, rather than historical fact?

    a. Leif Erikson was definitely the son of Erik the Red; however, historians debate the year of his birth.

    b. Leif Erikson's crew called the land Vinland since it was plentiful with grapes.

    c. Leif Erikson deserves more credit for his contributions in exploring the New World.

    d. Leif Erikson explored the Americas nearly five hundred years before Christopher Columbus.

Explanation

Answer. C: Choice *C* is the correct answer; it is the author's opinion that Erikson deserves more credit, not a verifiable fact.

Types of Writing

There are four main types of writing: narrative, expository, descriptive, and persuasive.

Narrative writing: When an author writes a narrative, they are telling a story. Narratives develop characters, drive a sequence of events, and deal with conflict. Examples of classic narratives are *The Great Gatsby*, *One Hundred Years of Solitude*, and *Song of Solomon*.

Expository writing: Expository writing is meant to instruct or inform and usually lacks any kind of persuasive elements. Expository writing includes recipes, academic lessons, repair manuals, or newspaper articles. Expository writing in academia uses third-person point of view and strives to be non-bias in its presentation.

Descriptive writing: Descriptive writing is writing that uses imagery and figurative language in order to allow the reader to feel as if they are experiencing the text firsthand. For example, a descriptive paragraph about Heather eating an ice cream cone will detail the smooth cream dripping down the cone, the crunch waffle, and the coldness and sweetness of the first bite. The reader is feeling the experience through the author's sensory language.

Persuasive writing: Persuasive writing is used when someone is writing an argument. Authors using persuasive writing are attempting to change the opinions and attitudes of their audience. Good persuasive writing will use credible sources and thoughtful analysis, stating both sides of the argument unbiasedly.

Example
Q. Which type of writing is meant to instruct of inform?
   a. Descriptive writing
   b. Narrative writing
   c. Persuasive writing
   d. Expository writing

Explanation
Answer. D: Expository writing is meant to instruct or inform. Expository writing does not tell a story, persuade the author, or rely only on descriptive language to get its point across.

Connotation and Denotation

The **connotative** meaning of a word is not the literal definition, but rather what the word implies. For example, the word *warm* literally means at a fair or comfortably high temperature. However, if I called a person *warm*, what does that imply? It implies they are friendly, welcoming, and comfortable around other people. Words can imply much more than their literal definitions.

The **denotative** meaning of a word is a word's literal definition, the one found in a dictionary. Students writing an academic paper will want to use words known for their strong denotative definitions rather than words associated with negative connotations.

Example
The question below is based on the following sentence.

Xavier *propagated* his belief that dragons were real to his friends gathered around the campfire.

Q. Which of the following words is the denotative form of the word *propagate?*
   a. Whispered
   b. Expressed
   c. Persuaded
   d. Shouted

<u>Explanation</u>
Answer. B: To *propagate* means to spread, disseminate, promote, or otherwise make known an idea, thought, or belief. The denotative form of a word is the literal definition of the word.

Author's Purpose

Author's write in order to persuade, entertain, inform, or express feelings. In reading comprehension exams, readers are tasked with the job of understanding the author's purpose for writing the passage. How can you tell what the author's purpose is? Let's look at a few scenarios below.

The author is writing to persuade: There is a clear argument in the passage. Furthermore, the author might ask the audience to take a stance or to act in some way.

The author is writing to entertain: The author is telling a story that entertains, like a narrative. There are characters that are going through a conflict, and there is a clear plot unfolding.

The author is writing to inform: There is information that the reader is expected to retain, like interesting facts or important statistics. A key difference between an informative author and a persuasive author is that the informative author will not take a side on a particular argument, nor will they ask their readers to.

The author is writing to express feelings: Many creative writers will write to express feelings. Look for certain word choices expressing love, sorrow, grief, happiness, or other strong emotions. Poetry contains many expressions of feeling. Writing to express feelings and writing to entertain are very similar, so choose the best answer choice you can with clues from the passage. Usually when authors write to express feelings, they use the first-person "I."

Example
Q. Which phrase best describes the purpose of nonfiction writing?
　　a. To inform, entertain, or persuade readers
　　b. To entertain, then to inform
　　c. To convince readers they're wrong about the author's subject
　　d. None of the above

Explanation
Answer. A: The correct answer is to inform, entertain, or persuade readers.

Author's Point of View

An author's **point-of-view** is the perspective from which the author writes. There are five different points of view. Let's look at them below.

First-person: First-person point of view uses the pronoun "I" to tell a story. The author may be referring to themselves, or they may be using a character separate from themselves to use first-person. First-person point of view can feel very personal since we are seeing the character's innermost thoughts.

Second-person: Second-person uses the pronoun "you." Second-person point-of-view is best used in documents like email or letters, when the audience is directly addressed.

Third-person limited: Third-person point-of-view uses the pronouns "he," "she," or "they." In this point-of-view, the audience knows the thoughts and actions of one single character.

Third-person omniscient: The word "omniscient" means "all-knowing," so in this point-of-view, the audience has access to the thoughts and feelings of all characters.

Third-person objective: In third-person objective, the audience has access to the characters' actions but does not have access to their thoughts and feelings.

Example

Q. Which of the following sentences uses second person point of view?

    a. I don't want to make plans for the weekend before I see my work schedule.

    b. She had to miss the last three yoga classes due to illness.

    c. Pluto is no longer considered a planet because it is not gravitationally dominant.

    d. Be sure to turn off all of the lights before locking up for the night.

Explanation

Answer. D: Choice *D* directly addresses the reader, so it is in second person point of view. This is an imperative sentence since it issues a command; imperative sentences have an *understood you* as the subject. Choice *A* uses first person pronouns *I* and *my*. Choices B and C are incorrect because they use third person point of view.

Using Text Features

Text features include bolding, italics, underlining, formatting, headings, and subheadings. Usually,

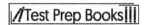

bolding words indicate key concepts, *italicizing* words indicate another language or an emphasis, and underlining can also indicate a key term.

Formatting can be anything from choosing left, center, and right justification, to keeping text together on a page. Researching proper ways to format is extremely helpful for writing theses, dissertations, books, or textbooks in general.

Headings and subheadings should be consistent with each other and should be used to organize information effectively.

<u>Example</u>

The next question is based on the following outline.

Chapter 5: Outdoor Activities

1. Hiking
   a. Gear
   b. First Aid
2. Camping
   a. Tents & Gear
   b. Camping Activities
3. Cycling
   a. Safety
   b. Finding Cycling Trails
4. Canoeing
   a. Equipment
   b. Tips for Maneuvering

Q. What aspect of this outline is inconsistent?

a. Hiking, which starts with an H, is included with activities that all start with C.

b. There is no information about gear/equipment for cycling

c. Rock climbing is not included in the outline.

d. There is no section for hiking tips.

<u>Explanation</u>

Answer. B: Choice *B* is the correct answer because every segment except cycling contains a section about equipment or gear.

Integration of Knowledge and Ideas

Primary Sources in Various Media

Primary sources are documents created during the time period which they reference. Examples of primary sources to use in research papers include government documents, photographs, speeches, journal entries, newspaper articles, or historical artifacts. Secondary sources are documents that analyze primary sources, such as websites, history books, or reviews.

Example
Q. First-hand accounts of an event, subject matter, time period, or an individual are referred to as what type of source?
- a. Primary sources
- b. Secondary sources
- c. Direct sources
- d. Indirect sources

Explanation
Answer. A: Firsthand accounts are given by primary sources—individuals who provide personal or expert accounts of an event, subject matter, time period, or of an individual.

Making Predictions and Drawing Conclusions

Predictions

Some texts use suspense and foreshadowing to captivate readers. For example, an intriguing aspect of murder mysteries is that the reader is never sure of the culprit until the author reveals the individual's identity. Authors often build suspense and add depth and meaning to a work by leaving clues to provide hints or predict future events in the story; this is called foreshadowing. While some instances of foreshadowing are subtle, others are quite obvious.

Conclusions

Active readers should also draw conclusions. When doing so, the reader should ask the following questions: What is this text about? What does the author believe? Does this text have merit? Do I believe the author? Would this text support my argument? Always read cautiously and critically. Interact with text, and record reactions in the margins. These active reading skills help determine the author's purpose as well as your own conclusion about the text.

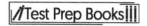

Example

Q. Which of the following statements would make the best conclusion to an essay about civil rights activist Rosa Parks?

> a. On December 1, 1955, Rosa Parks refused to give up her bus seat to a white passenger, setting in motion the Montgomery bus boycott.
> b. Rosa Parks was a hero to many and came to symbolize the way that ordinary people could bring about real change in the Civil Rights Movement.
> c. Rosa Parks died in 2005 in Detroit, having moved from Montgomery shortly after the bus boycott.
> d. Rosa Parks' arrest was an early part of the Civil Rights Movement and helped lead to the passage of the Civil Rights Act of 1964.

Explanation

Answer. B: Choice *A*, Choice *C*, and Choice *D* all relate facts but do not present the kind of general statement that would serve as an effective conclusion. Choice *B* is correct.

Theme or Central Message

The **theme** of a text is usually stated in one or two words and describes what the central message of a passage is. Themes like friendship, love, loss, coming-of-age, nature, loneliness, sacrifice, or pride are popular themes that people connect with on a deep level. Some themes are based in conflict, such as individual vs. nature, individual vs. society, or a hero archetype vs. a villain archetype.

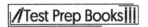

Example

Q. Read the following poem. Which option best expresses the symbolic meaning of the "road" and the overall theme?

> Two roads diverged in a yellow wood,
> And sorry I could not travel both
> And be one traveler, long I stood
> And looked down one as far as I could
> To where it bent in the undergrowth;
> Then took the other, as just as fair,
> And having perhaps the better claim,
> Because it was grassy and wanted wear;
> Though as for that the passing there
> Had worn them really about the same,
> And both that morning equally lay
> In leaves no step had trodden black.
> Oh, I kept the first for another day!
> Yet knowing how way leads on to way,
> I doubted if I should ever come back.
> I shall be telling this with a sigh
> Somewhere ages and ages hence:
> Two roads diverged in a wood, and I—
> I took the one less traveled by,
> And that has made all the difference—Robert Frost, "The Road Not Taken"

a. A divergent spot where the traveler had to choose the correct path to his destination
b. A choice between good and evil that the traveler needs to make
c. The traveler's struggle between his lost love and his future prospects
d. Life's journey and the choices with which humans are faced

Explanation

Answer. D: Choice *D* correctly summarizes Frost's theme of life's journey and the choices one makes. While Choice *A* can be seen as an interpretation, it is a literal one and is not the overall theme. Literal is not symbolic. Choice *B* presents the idea of good and evil as a theme, and the poem does not specify this struggle for the traveler. Choice *C* is a similarly incorrect answer. Love is not the theme.

Evaluating an Argument

The author's **credibility** is important to an argument; who is the author and what credentials do they have in relation to their topic? Is their writing clean, organized, and unbiased? The **evidence** an author uses must be credible as well; check where the sources came from. Is the date relevant, and are the sources from noteworthy articles or peer-reviewed journals? Next, what is the author using as their

appeal to emotion? Are they use pathos (emotion), logos (logic), or relying on ethos (credibility), or using all three in a balanced way? Finally, has the author presented any counterarguments to show the opposition's side? **Counterarguments** show that the author is nonbiased and has explored every avenue possible.

Example

Q. Which of these descriptions gives the most detailed and objective support for the claim that drinking and driving is unsafe?

a. A dramatized television commercial reenacting a fatal drinking and driving accident, including heart-wrenching testimonials from loved ones

b. The Department of Transportation's press release noting the additional drinking and driving special patrol units that will be on the road during the holiday season

c. Congressional written testimony on the number of drinking and driving incidents across the country and their relationship to underage drinking statistics, according to experts

d. A highway bulletin warning drivers of penalties associated with drinking and driving

Explanation

Answer. C: Choice *C* is the correct answer.

Mathematics

Numbers and Algebra

Conversions

<u>Decimals to Percentages</u>
To convert a percentage to a decimal, move the decimal point two places to the left and remove the % sign. To convert a decimal to a percentage, move the decimal point two places to the right and add a "%" sign. Here are some examples:

$$65\% = 0.65$$
$$0.33 = 33\%$$
$$0.215 = 21.5\%$$

<u>Fractions and Percentages</u>
A percentage can be converted to a fraction by making the number in the percentage the numerator and putting 100 as the denominator:

$$43\% = \frac{43}{100}$$
$$97\% = \frac{97}{100}$$

To convert a fraction to a percent, divide the numerator by the denominator to get a decimal:

$$\frac{9}{12} = 0.75$$

Then convert the decimal to a percentage:

$$0.75 = 75\%$$

Example

Q. Express the solution to the following problem in decimal form:

$$\frac{3}{5} \times \frac{7}{10} \div \frac{1}{2}$$

    a. 0.042
    b. 84%
    c. 0.84
    d. 0.42

Explanation

Answer. C: Separate this problem first by solving the division operation of the last two fractions. When dividing one fraction by another, invert or flip the second fraction and then multiply the numerator and denominator.

$$\frac{7}{10} \times \frac{2}{1} = \frac{14}{10}$$

Next, multiply the first fraction with this value:

$$\frac{3}{5} \times \frac{14}{10} = \frac{42}{50}$$

Decimals are expressions of 1 or 100%, so multiply both the numerator and denominator by 2 to get the fraction as an expression of 100.

$$\frac{42}{50} \times \frac{2}{2} = \frac{84}{100}$$

In decimal form, this would be expressed as 0.84.

Arithmetic Operations with Rational Numbers

Addition

Addition is the combination of two numbers so that their quantities are added together cumulatively. The sign for an addition operation is the $+$ symbol. For example, $9 + 6 = 15$. The 9 and 6 combine to achieve a cumulative value, called a sum.

Subtraction

Subtraction is taking away one number from another so that their quantities are reduced. The sign designating a subtraction operation is the $-$ symbol, and the result is called the difference. For example, $9 - 6 = 3$. The number *6* detracts from the number *9* to reach the difference *3*.

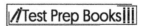

When working through subtraction problems involving larger numbers, it's necessary to regroup the numbers. Let's work through a practice problem using regrouping:

$$3\ 2\ 5$$
$$-\ 7\ 7$$

Here, it is clear that the ones and tens columns for 77 are greater than the ones and tens columns for 325. To subtract this number, borrow from the tens and hundreds columns. When borrowing from a column, subtracting 1 from the lender column will add 10 to the borrower column:

$$
\begin{array}{ccc}
3\text{-}1 & 10\text{+}2\text{-}1 & 10\text{+}5 \\
-\quad 7 & & 7 \\
\end{array}
=
\begin{array}{ccc}
2 & 11 & 15 \\
-\quad & 7 & 7 \\
\hline
2 & 4 & 8
\end{array}
$$

After ensuring that each digit in the top row is greater than the digit in the corresponding bottom row, subtraction can proceed as normal, and the answer is found to be 248.

Multiplication

Multiplication involves adding together multiple copies of a number. It is indicated by an × symbol or a number immediately outside of a parenthesis.

The two numbers being multiplied together are called factors, and their result is called a product. For example, $9 \times 6 = 54$. This can be shown alternatively by expansion of either the 9 or the 6:

$$9 \times 6 = 9 + 9 + 9 + 9 + 9 + 9 = 54$$

$$9 \times 6 = 6 + 6 + 6 + 6 + 6 + 6 + 6 + 6 + 6 = 54$$

Division

The signs designating a division operation are the ÷ and / symbols. In division, the second number divides into the first. The number before the division sign is called the dividend or, if expressed as a fraction, the numerator. For example, in $a \div b$, a is the dividend, while in $\frac{a}{b}$, a is the numerator. The number after the division sign is called the divisor or, if expressed as a fraction, the denominator. For example, in $a \div b$, b is the divisor, while in $\frac{a}{b}$, b is the denominator. If a divisor doesn't divide into a dividend an integer number of times, whatever is left over is termed the remainder.

Example

Q. What is the solution to $4 \times 7 + (25 - 21)^2 \div 2$?

   a. 512
   b. 36
   c. 60.5
   d. 22

Explanation

Answer. B: To solve this correctly, keep in mind the order of operations with the mnemonic PEMDAS (Please Excuse My Dear Aunt Sally). This stands for Parentheses, Exponents, Multiplication, Division, Addition, Subtraction. Taking it step by step, solve the parentheses first:

$$4 \times 7 + (4)^2 \div 2$$

Then, apply the exponent:

$$4 \times 7 + 16 \div 2$$

Multiplication and division are both performed next:

$$28 + 8 = 36$$

Comparing and Ordering Rational Numbers

A common question type asks to order rational numbers from least to greatest or greatest to least. The numbers will come in a variety of formats, including decimals, percentages, roots, fractions, and whole numbers.

Whether the question asks to order the numbers from greatest to least or least to greatest, the crux of the question is the same—convert the numbers into a common format. Generally, it's easiest to write the numbers as whole numbers and decimals so they can be placed on a number line.

Example

Q. Arrange the following numbers from least to greatest value:

$0.85, \frac{4}{5}, \frac{2}{3}, \frac{91}{100}$

a. $0.85, \frac{4}{5}, \frac{2}{3}, \frac{91}{100}$

b. $\frac{4}{5}, 0.85, \frac{91}{100}, \frac{2}{3}$

c. $\frac{2}{3}, \frac{4}{5}, 0.85, \frac{91}{100}$

d. $0.85, \frac{91}{100}, \frac{4}{5}, \frac{2}{3}$

Explanation

Answer. C: The first step is to depict each number using decimals. $\frac{91}{100}$ = 0.91

Dividing the numerator by denominator of $\frac{4}{5}$ to convert it to a decimal yields 0.80, while $\frac{2}{3}$ becomes 0.66 recurring. Rearrange each expression in ascending order, as found in answer C.

Solving Equations in One Variable

Solving equations in one variable is the process of isolating a variable on one side of the equation. *X* is commonly used as a variable, though any letter can be used.

Example
Q. What is the value of *b* in this equation?
$$5b - 4 = 2b + 17$$

a. 13
b. 24
c. 7
d. 21

Explanation
Answer. C: To solve for the value of b, both sides of the equation need to be equalized.

Start by cancelling out the lower value of -4 by adding 4 to both sides:

$$5b - 4 + 4 = 2b + 17 + 4$$

$$5b = 2b + 21$$

The variable *b* is the same on each side, so subtract the lower 2b from each side:

$$5b - 2b = 2b + 21 - 2b$$

$$3b = 21$$

Then divide both sides by 3 to get the value of *b*:

$$b = 7$$

Solving Multistep Problems with Rational Numbers

The key to answering word problems is to translate the words into a math problem. Always keep in mind what the question is asking and what operations could lead to that answer.

Example
Q. If Sarah reads at an average rate of 21 pages in four nights, how long will it take her to read 140 pages?
- a. 6 nights
- b. 26 nights
- c. 8 nights
- d. 27 nights

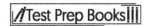

Explanation

Answer. D: This problem can be solved by setting up a proportion involving the given information and the unknown value. The proportion is:

$$\frac{21\ pages}{4\ nights} = \frac{140\ pages}{x\ nights}$$

Solving the proportion by cross-multiplying, the equation becomes $21x = 4 \times 140$, where $x = 26.67$. Since it is not an exact number of nights, the answer is rounded up to 27 nights. Twenty-six nights would not give Sarah enough time.

Solving Real World Problems Involving Percentages

Questions dealing with percentages almost always come in three varieties. The first type will ask to find what percentage of some number will equal another number. The second asks to determine what number is some percentage of another given number. The third will ask what number another number is a given percentage of.

Example

Q. A student gets an 85% on a test with 20 questions. How many answers did the student solve correctly?

  a. 15
  b. 16
  c. 17
  d. 18

Explanation

Answer. C: 85% of a number means that number should be multiplied by 0.85: $0.85 \times 20 = \frac{85}{100} \times \frac{20}{1}$, which can be simplified to $\frac{17}{20} \times \frac{20}{1} = 17$.

Estimation Strategies and Rounding Rules

Estimation

Estimation is finding a value that is close to a solution but is not the exact answer. For example, if there are values in the thousands to be multiplied, then each value can be estimated to the nearest thousand and the calculation performed.

Rounding Numbers

It's often convenient to **round a number**, which means to give an approximate figure to make it easier to compare amounts or perform mental math. Round up when the digit is 5 or more.

Reasonableness of Results
When solving math word problems, the solution obtained should make sense within the given scenario. The step of checking the solution will reduce the possibility of a calculation error or a solution that may be mathematically correct but not applicable in the real world.

Mental Math Estimation
Once a result is determined to be logical within the context of a given problem, the result should be evaluated by its nearness to the expected answer. This is performed by approximating given values to perform mental math. Numbers should be rounded to the nearest value possible to check the initial results.

Example
A customer is buying a new sound system for their home. The customer purchases a stereo for $435, 2 speakers for $67 each, and the necessary cables for $12. The customer chooses an option that allows him to spread the costs over equal payments for 4 months. How much will the monthly payments be?

Explanation
After making calculations for the problem, a student determines that the monthly payment will be $145.25. To check the accuracy of the results, the student rounds each cost to the nearest ten (440 + 70 + 70 +

10) and determines that the total is approximately $590. Dividing by 4 months gives an approximate monthly payment of $147.50. Therefore, the student can conclude that the solution of $145.25 is very close to what should be expected.

Solving Real World Problems Involving Proportions

Proportional reasoning can be used to solve problems involving ratios, percentages, and averages. Ratios can be used in setting up proportions and solving them to find unknowns. For example, if a student completes an average of 10 pages of math homework in 3 nights, how long would it take the student to complete 22 pages? Both ratios can be written as fractions. The second ratio would contain the unknown.

Example
Q. In Jim's school, there are 3 girls for every 2 boys. There are 650 students in total. Using this information, how many students are girls?

    a. 260
    b. 130
    c. 65
    d. 390

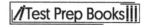

Explanation

Answer. D: Three girls for every two boys can be expressed as a ratio: 3:2. This can be visualized as splitting the school into 5 groups: 3 girl groups and 2 boy groups. The number of students who are in each group can be found by dividing the total number of students by 5:

650 divided by 5 equals 1 part, or 130 students per group.

To find the total number of girls, multiply the number of students per group (130) by the number of girl groups in the school (3). This equals 390, answer *D*.

Solving Real-World Problems Involving Ratios and Rates of Change

Ratios

Ratios are used to show the relationship between two quantities. The ratio of oranges to apples in the grocery store may be 3 to 2. That means that for every 3 oranges, there are 2 apples. This comparison can be expanded to represent the actual number of oranges and apples.

Unit Rate

Unit rates are the simplest form of rate. With unit rates, the denominator in the comparison of two units is one. For example, if someone can type at a rate of 1000 words in 5 minutes, then his or her unit rate for typing is $\frac{1000}{5} = 200$ words in one minute or 200 words per minute.

Rate of Change

Rate of change for any line calculates the steepness of the line over a given interval. Rate of change is also known as the slope, or $\frac{rise}{run}$. The TEAS will focus on the rate of change for linear functions which are straight lines. The slope is given by the change in y divided by the change in x.

So, the formula looks like this:

$$slope = \frac{y_2 - y_1}{x_2 - x_1}$$

Example
The following question is based on the image below.

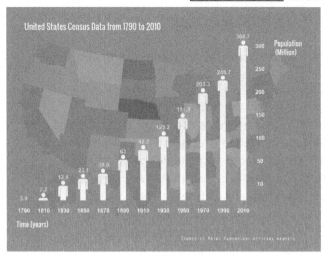

United States Census Data from 1790 to 2010

Q. In what year did the population increase the most during a twenty-year interval?

    a. From 1930 to 1950

    b. From 1950 to 1970

    c. From 1970 to 1990

    d. From 1990 to 2010

Explanation

Answer. D: The population increased the most between 1990 and 2010.

Measurement and Data

Information from Tables, Charts, and Graphs

Tables

One of the most common ways to express data is in a **table**. The primary reason for plugging data into a table is to make interpretation more convenient. It's much easier to look at the table than to analyze results in a narrative paragraph. When analyzing a table, pay close attention to the title, variables, and data.

Results of Antibiotic Studies		
Group	**Dosage of Antibiotics in milligrams (mg)**	**Efficacy (% of participants cured)**
A	0 mg	20%
B	20 mg	40%
C	40 mg	75%
D	60 mg	95%
E	80 mg	100%
F	100 mg	100%

Charts

Chart is a broad term that refers to a variety of ways to represent data.

To graph relations, the **Cartesian plane** is used. This means to think of the plane as being given a grid of squares, with one direction being the *x*-axis and the other direction the *y*-axis.

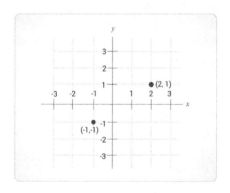

Graphs

Graphs provide a visual representation of data. The variables are placed on the two axes. The bottom of the graph is referred to as the horizontal axis or X-axis. The left-hand side of the graph is known as the vertical axis or Y-axis. Typically, the independent variable is placed on the X-axis, and the dependent variable is located on the Y-axis.

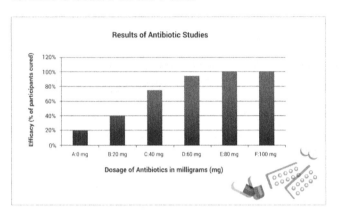

Example

Q. The following graph compares the various test scores of the top three students in each of these teacher's classes. Based on the graph, which teacher's students had the lowest range of test scores?

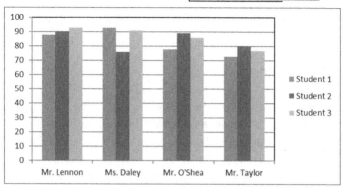

a. Mr. Lennon
b. Mr. O'Shea
c. Mr. Taylor
d. Ms. Daley

Explanation

Answer. A: To calculate the range in a set of data, subtract the highest value with the lowest value. In this graph, the range of Mr. Lennon's students is 5, which can be seen physically in the graph as having the smallest difference compared with the other teachers between the highest value and the lowest value.

Information in Tables, Charts, and Graphs Using Statistics

Mean, Median, and Mode

The center of a set of data can be represented by its mean, median, or mode. These are sometimes referred to as **measures of central tendency**. The **mean** is the average. To find the mean, add up all the data points, then divide by the total number of data points. In a data set, the **median** is the point in the middle. The middle refers to the point where half the data comes before it and half comes after, when the data is recorded in numerical order. One additional measure to define for X is the **mode**. This is the data point that appears most frequently. If two or more data points all tie for the most frequent appearance, then each of them is considered a mode.

Set of Data

A **set of data** can be described in terms of its center, spread, shape and any unusual features. The center of a data set can be measured by its mean, median, or mode. The spread of a data set refers to how far the data points are from the center (mean or median). A data set with data points clustered around the center will have a small spread. A data set covering a wide range will have a large spread.

Correlation

An **X-Y diagram**, also known as a scatter diagram, visually displays the relationship between two variables. The independent variable is placed on the x-axis, and the dependent variable is placed on the y-axis.

Example

Q. What is the overall median of Dwayne's current scores: 78, 92, 83, 97?

    a. 19
    b. 85
    c. 83
    d. 87.5

Explanation

Answer. D: For an even number of total values, the median is calculated by finding the mean or average of the two middle values once all values have been arranged in ascending order from least to greatest. In this case, $(92 + 83) \div 2$ would equal the median 87.5, answer *D*.

Relationship Between Two Variables

In an experiment, variables are the key to analyzing data. Variables can represent anything, including objects, conditions, events, and amounts of time.

Covariance is a general term referring to how two variables move in relation to each other.

Constant variables remain unchanged by the scientist across all trials.

Independent variables are also controlled by the scientist, but they are the same only for each group or trial in the experiment.

Dependent variables experience change caused by the independent variable and are what is being measured or observed.

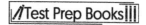

Example

Q. In testing how quickly a rat dies by the amount of poison it eats, which of the following is the independent variable and which is the dependent variable?

    a. How quickly the rat dies is the independent variable; the amount of poison is the dependent variable.

    b. The amount of poison is the independent variable; how quickly the rat dies is the dependent variable.

    c. Whether the rat eats the poison is the independent variable; how quickly the rat dies is the dependent variable.

    d. The cage the rat is kept in is the independent variable; the amount of poison is the dependent variable.

Explanation

Answer. B: The independent variable is the variable manipulated and the dependent variable is the result of the changes in the independent variable. Choice *B* is correct because the amount of poison is the variable that is changed, and the speed of rat death is the result of the changes in the amount of poison administered.

Calculating Geometric Quantities

Perimeter

Perimeter is the measurement of a distance around something or the sum of all sides of a polygon. Formulas for measuring perimeters are below.

    A.   Square: $P = 4 \times s$
    B.   Rectangle: $P = l + l + w + w = 2l + 2w$
    C.   Triangle: $P = a + b + c$
    D.   Circle: $\pi \times d$

Area

Area in mathematics is defined as the space occupied by an object. Below are various area formulas.

    E.   Square: $A = s^2$
    F.   Rectangle: $A = l \times w$
    G.   Triangle: $A = \dfrac{bh}{2}$
    H.   Circle: $A = \pi \times r^2$

Arc

The **arc of a circle** is the distance between two points on the circle. The length of the arc of a circle in terms of degrees is easily determined if the value of the central angle is known. The length of the arc is simply the value of the central angle. In this example, the length of the arc of the circle in degrees is 75°.

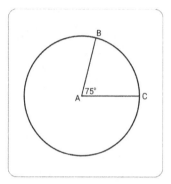

To determine the length of the arc of a circle in distance, the student will need to know the values for both the central angle and the radius. This formula is:

$$\frac{central\ angle}{360°} = \frac{arc\ length}{2\pi r}$$

The equation is simplified by cross-multiplying to solve for the arc length.

Irregular Shapes

The perimeter of an irregular polygon is found by adding the lengths of all of the sides. In cases where all of the sides are given, this will be very straightforward. Other times, a side length may be missing and must be determined before the perimeter can be calculated.

Example

Q. The total perimeter of a rectangle is 36 cm. If the length of each side is 12 cm, what is the width?

    a. 3 cm

    b. 12 cm

    c. 6 cm

    d. 8 cm

Explanation

Answer. C: The first step is to substitute all of the data into the formula:

$$36 = 2(12) + 2W$$

Simplify by multiplying 2×12:

$$36 = 24 + 2W$$

Simplifying this further by subtracting 24 on each side, which gives:

$$36 - 24 = 24 - 24 + 2W$$

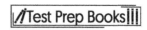

$$12 = 2W$$

Divide by 2:

$$6 = W$$

Standard and Metric Systems

<u>American Measuring System</u>
The measuring system used today in the United States developed from the British units of measurement during colonial times. The most typically used units in this customary system are those used to measure weight, liquid volume, and length, whose common units are found below.

Common Customary Measurements		
Length	**Weight**	**Capacity**
1 foot = 12 inches	1 pound = 16 ounces	1 cup = 8 fluid ounces
1 yard = 3 feet	1 ton = 2,000 pounds	1 pint = 2 cups
1 yard = 36 inches		1 quart = 2 pints
1 mile = 1,760 yards		1 quart = 4 cups
1 mile = 5,280 feet		1 gallon = 4 quarts
		1 gallon = 16 cups

Metric System

Aside from the United States, most countries in the world have adopted the metric system embodied in the International System of Units (SI). The three main SI base units used in the metric system are the meter (m), the kilogram (kg), and the liter (L); meters measure length, kilograms measure mass, and liters measure volume.

These three units can use different prefixes, which indicate larger or smaller versions of the unit by powers of ten. This can be thought of as making a new unit which is sized by multiplying the original unit in size by a factor.

These prefixes and associated factors are:

Metric Prefixes			
Prefix	Symbol	Multiplier	Exponential
kilo	k	1,000	10^3
hecto	h	100	10^2
deca	da	10	10^1
no prefix		1	10^0
deci	d	0.1	10^{-1}
centi	c	0.01	10^{-2}
milli	m	0.001	10^{-3}

Conversion

Converting measurements in different units between the two systems can be difficult because they follow different rules. The table below lists some common conversion values that are useful for problems involving measurements with units in both systems:

English System	Metric System
1 inch	2.54 cm
1 foot	0.3048 m
1 yard	0.914 m
1 mile	1.609 km
1 ounce	28.35 g
1 pound	0.454 kg
1 fluid ounce	29.574 mL
1 quart	0.946 L
1 gallon	3.785 L

Example

Q. Mom's car drove 72 miles in 90 minutes. How fast did she drive in feet per second?

    a. 0.8 feet per second
    b. 48.9 feet per second
    c. 0.009 feet per second
    d. 70. 4 feet per second

Explanation

Answer. D: This problem can be solved by using unit conversions. The initial units are miles per minute. The final units need to be feet per second. Converting miles to feet uses the equivalence statement 1 mile = 5,280 feet. Converting minutes to seconds uses the equivalence statement 1 minute = 60 seconds. Setting up the ratios to convert the units is shown in the following equation: $\frac{72\ miles}{90\ minutes} \times \frac{1\ minute}{60\ seconds} \times \frac{5280\ feet}{1\ mile} = 70.4$ feet per second. The initial units cancel out, and the new, desired units are left.

Science

General Anatomy and Physiology of a Human

Anatomy may be defined as the structural makeup of an organism. **Physiology** refers to the functions of an organism and it examines the chemical or physical functions that help the body function appropriately.

Levels of Organization of the Human Body
All the parts of the human body are built of individual units called **cells**. Groups of similar cells are arranged into **tissues**, different tissues are arranged into **organs**, and organs working together form entire **organ systems**. The human body has twelve organ systems that govern circulation, digestion, immunity, hormones, movement, support, coordination, urination & excretion, reproduction (male and female), respiration, and general protection.

Body Cavities
The body is partitioned into different hollow spaces that house organs. The human body contains the following **cavities**:

- Cranial cavity
- Thoracic cavity
- Abdominal cavity

- Pelvic cavity
- Spinal cavity

Human Tissues

Human tissues can be grouped into four categories:

I. Muscle
J. Nervous
K. Epithelial
L. Connective

Three Primary Body Planes

A plane is an imaginary flat surface. The three primary planes of the human body are frontal, sagittal, and transverse.

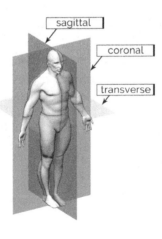

Terms of Direction

M. **Medial** refers to a structure being closer to the midline of the body.

N. **Lateral** refers to a structure being farther from the midline of the body, and it is the opposite of medial.

O. **Proximal** refers to a structure or body part located near an attachment point.

P. **Distal** refers to a structure or body part located far from an attachment point.

Q. **Anterior** means toward the front in humans.

R. **Posterior** means toward the back in humans.

S. **Superior** means above and refers to a structure closer to the head.

T. **Inferior** means below and refers to a structure farther from the head.

U. **Superficial** refers to a structure closer to the surface.

V. **Deep** refers to a structure farther from the surface.

Body Regions

Terms for general locations on the body include:

W. Cervical: relating to the neck

X. Clavicular: relating to the clavicle

Y. Ocular: relating to the eyes

Z. Acromial: relating to the shoulder

AA. Cubital: relating to the elbow

BB. Brachial: relating to the arm

CC. Carpal: relating to the wrist

DD. Thoracic : relating to the chest

EE. Abdominal: relating to the abdomen

FF. Pubic: relating to the groin

GG. Pelvic: relating to the pelvis

HH. Femoral: relating to the femur, or thigh bone

II. Geniculate: relating to the knee

JJ. Pedal: relating to the foot

KK. Palmar: relating to the palm of the hand

LL. Plantar: relating to the sole of the foot

Abdominopelvic Regions and Quadrants

The **abdominopelvic region** may be defined as the combination of the abdominal and the pelvic cavities. The region's upper border is the breasts and its lower border is the groin region.

A simple way to describe the abdominopelvic area would be to divide it into the following quadrants:

MM.　　　Right upper quadrant (RUQ): Encompasses the right hypochondriac, right lumbar, epigastric, and umbilical regions.

NN. Right lower quadrant (RLQ): Encompasses the right lumbar, right inguinal, hypogastric, and umbilical regions.

OO. Left upper quadrant (LUQ): Encompasses the left hypochondriac, left lumbar, epigastric, and umbilical regions.
PP. Left lower quadrant (LLQ): Encompasses the left lumbar, left inguinal, hypogastric, and umbilical regions.

Cell Structure and Function
The **cell** is the main functional and structural component of all living organisms. The cell theory is composed of three principals:

QQ. 1. All organisms are composed of cells.
RR. 2. All existing cells are created from other living cells.
SS. 3. The cell is the most fundamental unit of life.

Organisms can be unicellular (composed of one cell) or multicellular (composed of many cells). All cells must be bounded by a cell membrane, be filled with cytoplasm of some sort, and be coded by a genetic sequence.

Prokaryotes and Eukaryotes
The majority of **prokaryotic** cells have cell walls, while most **eukaryotic** cells do not have cell walls. The DNA of prokaryotic cells is contained in a single circular chromosome, while the DNA of eukaryotic cells is contained in multiple linear chromosomes.

Prokaryotic cells divide using binary fission, while eukaryotic cells divide using mitosis. Examples of prokaryotes are bacteria and archaea while examples of eukaryotes are animals and plants.

Nuclear Parts of a Cell

TT. Nucleus: Houses a cell's genetic material, deoxyribonucleic acid (DNA)

UU. Chromosomes: Complex thread-like arrangements composed of DNA found in a cell's nucleus.

VV. Chromatin: An aggregate of genetic material consisting of DNA and proteins that forms chromosomes during cell division.

WW.   Nucleolus: The largest component of the nucleus of a eukaryotic cell.

Cell Membranes

Cell membranes encircle the cell's cytoplasm, separating the intracellular environment from the extracellular environment. They are selectively permeable, which enables them to control molecular traffic entering and exiting cells.

Passive Transport Mechanisms

Passive transport refers to the migration of molecules across a cell membrane that does not require energy. The three types of passive transport include simple diffusion, facilitated diffusion, and osmosis.

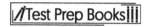

Simple diffusion relies on a concentration gradient, or differing quantities of molecules inside or outside of a cell. **Facilitated diffusion** utilizes carrier proteins to transport molecules across a cell membrane. **Osmosis** refers to the transport of water across a selectively permeable membrane.

Active Transport Mechanisms
Active transport refers to the migration of molecules across a cell membrane that requires energy. It's a useful way to move molecules from an area of low concentration to an area of high concentration. Adenosine triphosphate (ATP), the currency of cellular energy, is needed to work against the concentration gradient.

Structure and Function of Cellular Organelles
Organelles are specialized structures that perform specific tasks in a cell. The term literally means "little organ." Most organelles are membrane bound and serve as sites for the production or degradation of chemicals.

Here an illustration of the cell:

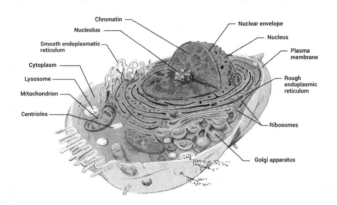

Example

Q. Using anatomical terms, what is the relationship of the sternum relative to the deltoid?

    a. Medial

    b. Lateral

    c. Superficial

    d. Posterior

Explanation

Answer. A: The sternum is medial to the deltoid because it is much closer (typically right on) the midline of the body, while the deltoid is lateral at the shoulder cap. Superficial means that a structure is closer to the body surface and posterior means that it falls behind something else. For example, skin is superficial to bone and the kidneys are posterior to the rectus abdominus.

Respiratory System

The respiratory system enables breathing and supports the energy-making process in our cells. The respiratory system transports an essential reactant, oxygen, to cells so that they can produce energy in their mitochondria via cellular respiration. The respiratory system also removes carbon dioxide, a waste product of cellular respiration.

Example
Q. Which of the following is NOT a major function of the respiratory system in humans?

a. It provides a large surface area for gas exchange of oxygen and carbon dioxide.
b. It helps regulate the blood's pH.
c. It helps cushion the heart against jarring motions.
d. It is responsible for vocalization.

Explanation
Answer. C: Although the lungs may provide some cushioning for the heart when the body is violently struck, this is not a major function of the respiratory system.

Cardiovascular System

The cardiovascular system (also called the circulatory system) is a network of organs and tubes that transport blood, hormones, nutrients, oxygen, and other gases to cells and tissues throughout the body. The major components of the circulatory system are the blood vessels, blood, and heart.

Example
Q. What type of vessel carries oxygen-rich blood from the heart to other tissues of the body?
   a. Veins
   b. Intestines
   c. Bronchioles
   d. Arteries

Explanation
Answer. D: Arteries carry oxygen-rich blood from the heart to the other tissues of the body. Veins carry oxygen-poor blood back to the heart. Intestines carry digested food through the body. Bronchioles are passageways that carry air from the nose and mouth to the lungs.

Gastrointestinal System

The human body relies completely on the digestive system to meet its nutritional needs. After food and drink are ingested, the digestive system breaks them down into their component nutrients and absorbs them so that the circulatory system can transport them to other cells to use for growth, energy, and cell repair. These nutrients may be classified as proteins, lipids, carbohydrates, vitamins, and minerals.

Example
Q. Which locations in the digestive system are sites of chemical digestion?

> I. Mouth
> II. Stomach
> III. Small Intestine

a. II only
b. III only
c. II and III only
d. I, II, and III

Explanation
Answer. D: Chemical digestion involves chemically changing the food and breaking it down into small organic compounds that can be utilized by the cell to build molecules. The salivary glands in the mouth secrete amylase that breaks down starch, which begins chemical digestion. The stomach contains enzymes such as pepsinogen/pepsin and gastric lipase, which chemically digest protein and fats. The small

intestine continues to digest protein using the enzymes trypsin and chymotrypsin

Neuromuscular System

The human nervous system coordinates the body's response to stimuli from inside and outside the body. There are two major types of nervous system cells: neurons and neuroglia. Neurons are the workhorses of the nervous system and form a complex communication network that transmits electrical impulses termed action potentials, while neuroglia connect and support them.

Example
Q. How many neurons generally make up a sensory pathway?

    a. 1
    b. 2
    c. 3
    d. 4

Explanation
Answer. C: Generally, all sensory pathways that extend from the sensory receptor to the brain are composed of three long neurons called the primary, secondary, and tertiary neurons. The primary one stretches from the sensory receptor to the dorsal root ganglion of the spinal nerve; the secondary one

stretches from the cell body of the primary neuron to the spinal cord or the brain stem; the tertiary one stretches from the cell body of the secondary one into the thalamus.

Reproductive System

The reproductive system is responsible for producing, storing, nourishing, and transporting functional reproductive cells, or gametes, in the human body. It includes the reproductive organs, also known as gonads, the reproductive tract, the accessory glands and organs that secrete fluids into the reproductive tract, and the perineal structures, which are the external genitalia.

Example
Q. Where does sperm maturation take place in the male reproductive system?
 a. Seminal vesicles
 b. Prostate gland
 c. Epididymis
 d. Vas Deferens

Explanation
Answer. C: The epididymis stores sperm and is a coiled tube located near the testes.

Integumentary System

The integumentary system includes skin, hair, nails, oil glands, and sweat glands. The largest organ of the integumentary system (and of the body), the skin, acts as a barrier and protects the body from mechanical impact, variations in temperature, microorganisms, chemicals, and UV radiation from the sun. It regulates body temperature, peripheral circulation, and excretes waste through sweat. It also contains a large network of nerve cells that relay changes in the external environment to the brain.

Example
Q. Which of the following areas of the body has the most sweat glands?

    a. Upper back
    b. Arms
    c. Feet
    d. Palms

Explanation
Answer. A: The upper back has the one of the high densities of sweat glands of any area on the body.

Endocrine System

The endocrine system is made up of the ductless tissues and glands that secrete hormones directly into the bloodstream. It is similar to the nervous system in that it controls various functions of the body, but it does so via secretion of hormones in the bloodstream as opposed to nerve impulses. The endocrine system is also different because its effects last longer than that of the nervous system. Nerve impulses are immediate while hormone responses can last for minutes or even days.

Example

Q. The primary function of the endocrine system is to maintain which of the following?

- a. Heartbeat
- b. Respiration
- c. Electrolyte and water balance
- d. Homeostasis

Explanation

Answer. D: The primary function of the endocrine system is to maintain homeostasis, which means it makes constant adjustments to the body's systemic physiology to maintain a stable internal environment.

Genitourinary System

The urinary system is made up of the kidneys, ureters, urinary bladder, and the urethra. It is the system responsible for removing waste products and balancing water and electrolyte concentrations in the blood. The urinary system has many important functions related to waste excretion. It regulates the concentrations of sodium, potassium, chloride, calcium, and other ions in the filtrate by controlling the amount of each that is reabsorbed during filtration.

Example

Q. Which of the following are functions of the urinary system?

> I. Synthesizing calcitriol and secreting erythropoietin
> II. Regulating the concentrations of sodium, potassium, chloride, calcium, and other ions
> III. Reabsorbing or secreting hydrogen ions and bicarbonate
> IV. Detecting reductions in blood volume and pressure

a. I, II, and III
b. II and III
c. II, III, and IV
d. All of the above

Explanation

Answer. D: The urinary system has many functions, the primary of which is removing waste products and balancing water and electrolyte concentrations in the blood. It also plays a key role in regulating ion concentrations, such as sodium, potassium, chloride, and calcium, in the filtrate. The urinary system helps maintain blood pH by reabsorbing or secreting hydrogen ions and bicarbonate as necessary. Certain kidney cells can detect reductions in blood volume and pressure and then can secrete renin to activate a hormone that causes increased reabsorption of sodium ions and water.

Immune System

The immune system is the body's defense against invading microorganisms (bacteria, viruses, fungi, and parasites) and other harmful, foreign substances. It is capable of limiting or preventing infection.

Example
Q. Which is the first event to happen in a primary immune response?

a. Macrophages phagocytose pathogens and present their antigens.
b. Neutrophils aggregate and act as cytotoxic, nonspecific killers of pathogens.
c. B lymphocytes make pathogen-specific antibodies.
d. Helper T cells secrete interleukins to activate pathogen-fighting cells.

Explanation

Answer. A: The first event that happens in a primary immune response is that macrophages ingest pathogens and display their antigens. Then, they secrete interleukin 1 to recruit helper T cells. Once helper T cells are activated, they secrete interleukin 2 to simulate plasma B and killer T cell production. Only then can plasma B make the pathogen specific antibodies.

Skeletal System

The skeletal system is composed of 206 bones interconnected by tough connective tissue called ligaments. The axial skeleton can be considered the north-south axis of the skeleton. It includes the spinal column, sternum, ribs, and skull. There are eighty bones in the axial skeleton, and thirty-three of them are vertebrae. The ribs make up twelve of the bones in the axial skeleton.

Example

Q. What makes bone resistant to shattering?

    a. The calcium salts deposited in the bone

    b. The collagen fibers

    c. The bone marrow and network of blood vessels

    d. The intricate balance of minerals and collagen fibers

Explanation

Answer. D: Bony matrix is an intricate lattice of collagen fibers and mineral salts, particularly calcium and phosphorus. The mineral salts are strong but brittle, and the collagen fibers are weak but flexible, so the combination of the two makes bone resistant to shattering and able to withstand the normal forces applied to it.

Life and Physical Sciences

Basic Macromolecules in a Biological System

Carbohydrates

Carbohydrates are sweet, ring-like sugar molecules that are built from carbon (carbo-) and oxygen & hydrogen (-hydrates, meaning water). They can exist as one-ring monosaccharides, like glucose, fructose, and galactose, or as two-ring disaccharides, like lactose, maltose, and sucrose. These simple sugars can be easily broken down and used via glycolysis to provide a source of quick energy. Polysaccharides are repeating chains of monosaccharide rings. They are more complex carbohydrates, and there are several types.

Proteins

Proteins are made from a combination of twenty amino acids. The varying amino acids are linked by peptide bonds and form the primary structure of the polypeptide, or chain of amino acids. The primary structure is the string of amino acids. It is the secondary, tertiary, and quaternary structure that determines protein shape and function.

Lipids

Lipids are mostly nonpolar, hydrophobic molecules that are not soluble in water. Triglycerides are a type of lipid with a glycerol backbone attached to three long fatty acid chains. These energy-storage molecules can exist as saturated fats or unsaturated fats.

Phospholipids are also composed of glycerol except they have two fatty acid tails. The third tail is replaced with a hydrophilic phosphate group. The amphipathic nature of this molecule results in a lipid bilayer where the "water-loving" hydrophilic heads face the extracellular matrix and cytoplasm and the "water-hating" hydrophobic tails face each other on the inside.

Steroids are another type of lipid. Cholesterol is a steroid that embeds itself in animal cell membranes and acts as a fluidity buffer. Steroid hormones such as testosterone and estrogen are responsible for transcriptional regulation in certain cells.

is a motor protein because it is involved in the process of muscle contraction.

Example
Q. Which of the following correctly matches a category of protein with a physiologic example?
a. Keratin is a structural protein
b. Antigens are hormonal proteins
c. Channel proteins are marker proteins
d. Actin is a transport protein

Explanation
Answer. A: Keratin is a structural protein and it is the primary constituent of things like hair and nails.

Chromosomes, Genes, and DNA

Nucleic Acids
Nucleic acids have two important duties in the body. As monomers, they are crucial for energy transfer. As polymers, they are a fundamental component of genetic material. Monomers are the simplest form of a biochemical, while polymers are the complex form of a biochemical.

Codons

A codon represents a sequence of three nucleotides, which codes for either one specific amino acid or a stop signal during protein synthesis. Codons are found on messenger RNA (mRNA).

RNA

Ribonucleic acid (RNA) plays crucial roles in protein synthesis and gene regulation. RNA is made of nucleotides consisting of ribose (a sugar), a phosphate group, and one of four possible nitrogen bases— adenine (A), cytosine (C), guanine (G), and uracil (U). RNA utilizes the nitrogen base uracil in place of the base thymine found in DNA. Another difference between RNA and DNA is that RNA is typically found as a single-stranded structure, while DNA typically exists in a double-stranded structure.

DNA

Deoxyribonucleic acid, or DNA, contains the genetic material that is passed from parent to offspring. It contains specific instructions for the development and function of a unique eukaryotic organism. The great majority of cells in a eukaryotic organism contains the same DNA.

Transcription

Transcription refers to a portion of DNA being copied into RNA, specifically mRNA. It represents the first

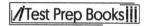

crucial step in gene expression. The process begins with the enzyme RNA polymerase binding to the promoter region of DNA, which initiates transcription of a specific gene. RNA polymerase then untwists the double helix of DNA by breaking weak hydrogen bonds between its nucleotides. Once DNA is untwisted, RNA polymerase travels down the strand reading the DNA sequence and adding complementary nitrogen bases. With the assistance of RNA polymerase, the pentose sugar and phosphate functional group are added to the nitrogen base to form a nucleotide. Lastly, the weak hydrogen bonds uniting the DNA-RNA complex are broken to free the newly formed mRNA. The mRNA travels from the nucleus of the cell out to the cytoplasm of the cell where translation occurs.

Translation
Translation refers to the process of ribosomes synthesizing proteins. It represents the second crucial step in gene expression. The instructions encoding specific proteins to be made are contained in codons on mRNA, which have previously been transcribed from DNA. Each codon represents a specific amino acid or stop signal in the genetic code.

Example

Q. Which of the following is directly transcribed from DNA and represents the first step in protein building?

    a. siRNA

    b. rRNA

    c. mRNA

    d. tRNA

Explanation

Answer. C: mRNA is directly transcribed from DNA before being taken to the cytoplasm and translated by rRNA into a protein. tRNA transfers amino acids from the cytoplasm to the rRNA for use in building these proteins. siRNA is a special type of RNA which interferes with other strands of mRNA typically by causing them to get degraded by the cell rather than translated into protein.

Mendel's Laws of Heredity

Genes are the basis of heredity. The German scientist Gregor Mendel first suggested the existence of genes in 1866. A gene can be pinpointed to a locus, or a particular position, on DNA. It is estimated that humans have approximately 20,000 to 25,000 genes. For any particular gene, a human inherits one copy from each parent for a total of two.

Genotype refers to the genetic makeup of an individual within a species. Phenotype refers to the visible characteristics and observable behavior of an individual within a species.

Mendel's first law of genetics is the principle of **segregation** and states that alleles will segregate into different cells during the formation of gametes in meiosis. Mendel's second law of genetics is the principle of **independent assortment** and states that genes for different traits will be assigned to different gametes independent of the others. Together, these two laws state the assumptions on which genetic probabilities are based.

Example

Q. What information does a genotype give that a phenotype does not?

  a. The genotype necessarily includes the proteins coded for by its alleles.

  b. The genotype will always show an organism's recessive alleles.

  c. The genotype must include the organism's physical characteristics.

  d. The genotype shows what an organism's parents looked like.

	T	t
T		
t		

Explanation

Answer. B: Since the genotype is a depiction of the specific alleles that an organism's genes code for, it includes recessive genes that may or may not be otherwise expressed.

Basic Atomic Structure

Measurable Properties of Atoms

All matter is made of atoms. **Atoms** are the most basic portion of an element that still retains its properties.

All of the elements known to man are catalogued in the periodic table, a chart of elements arranged by increasing atomic number. The atomic number refers to the number of protons in an atom's nucleus.

Periodicity and the Periodic Table

Periodicity refers to the repeating patterns, or trends, in the properties of elements. The atomic number and atomic structure are the key determinants of the properties of elements.

The **periodic table** catalogues all of the elements known to man, currently 118. It is one of the most important references in the science of chemistry. Information that can be gathered from the periodic table includes the element's atomic number, atomic mass, and chemical symbol.

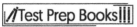

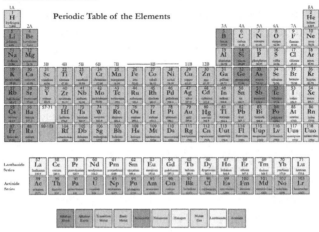

Ionic Bonding

Ionic bonds are formed from the electrostatic attractions between oppositely charged atoms. They result from the transfer of electrons from a metal on the left side of the periodic table to a nonmetal on the right side. In an ionic bond, an atom loses one or more electrons to another who gains them. The atoms do this so that they can achieve a full outermost shell of electrons, which is the configuration with the lowest amount of energy, and these are typically the strongest types of bonds.

Covalent Bonding

Covalent bonds are formed when two atoms share electrons, instead of transferring them like in ionic

96

compounds. The atoms in covalent compounds have a balance of attraction and repulsion between their protons and electrons, which keeps them bonded together. Two atoms can be joined by single, double, or even triple covalent bonds. As the number of electrons that are shared increases, the length of the bond decreases. Covalent substances have low melting and boiling points and are also poor conductors of heat and electricity. The Lewis structure for Cl_2 is written as follows:

$$\cdot \ddot{C}\ddot{l} \colon + \cdot \ddot{C}\ddot{l} \colon \rightarrow \colon \ddot{C}\ddot{l} \colon \ddot{C}\ddot{l} \colon$$

Hydrogen Bonding

Hydrogen bonds are temporary and weak. They typically occur between two partial, opposite electrical charges. For example, hydrogen bonds form when a hydrogen (H) atom in the vicinity of nitrogen (N), fluorine (F), or oxygen (O) atoms. These partial electrical charges are called **dipoles** and are caused by the unequal sharing of electrons between covalent bonds. Water is the most prevalent molecule that forms hydrogen bonds.

Metallic Bonds

Metallic bonds are formed by electrons that move freely through the metal. They are the product of the force of attraction between electrons and metal ions.

The electrons are shared by many metal cations and act like glue holding the metallic substance together. Metallic compounds have characteristic properties including strength, conduction of heat and electricity, and malleability. They can conduct electricity by passing energy through the freely moving electrons, creating a current. These compounds also have high melting and boiling points.

Example

Q. Salts like sodium iodide (NaI) and potassium chloride (KCl) use what type of bond?

    a. Ionic bonds

    b. Disulfide bridges

    c. Covalent bonds

    d. London dispersion forces

Explanation

Answer. A: Salts are formed from compounds that use ionic bonds.

Characteristic Properties of Substances

Properties of Water

Water is the most abundant substance on Earth. It is a compound composed of hydrogen and oxygen with the chemical formula H_2O. Water is also **polar**, which means it is negatively charged at one end and positively charged at the other end. The oxygen is more **electronegative** than the hydrogens, meaning that its protons pull in more of the electrons than do the hydrogens. This leaves the oxygen with a partial negative charge and the hydrogens with a partial positive charge.

Properties of Molecules
Molecules have both physical and chemical properties. Physical properties describe a substance in isolation, while chemical properties describe how a substance reacts with others. There are two types of physical properties: extensive and intensive. **Extensive physical properties** depend on the amount of a substance. Volume, length, and mass are all examples of extensive properties. **Intensive physical properties** are static and unchanging properties of a substance that identify it.

Example
Q. Which of the following is a special property of water?

a. Water easily flows through phospholipid bilayers.
b. A water molecule's oxygen atom allows fish to breathe.
c. Water is highly cohesive which explains its high melting point.
d. Water can self-hydrolyze and decompose into hydrogen and oxygen.

Explanation

Answer. C: Water's polarity lends it to be extremely cohesive and adhesive; this cohesion keeps its atoms very close together. Because of this, it takes a large amount of energy to melt and boil its solid and liquid forms.

States of Matter

Liquid

The molecules in a **liquid** are not in an orderly arrangement and can move past one another. Weak intermolecular forces contribute to a liquid having an indefinite shape, but definite volume. Lastly, a liquid conforms to the shape of its container, is not easily compressible, and flows quite easily.

Gas

The molecules in a **gas** have a large amount of space between them. A gas will diffuse indefinitely if unconfined, while it will assume the shape and volume of its container if enclosed. In other words, a gas has no definite shape or volume. Lastly, a gas is compressible and flows quite easily.

Solid

The molecules in a **solid** are closely packed together, which restricts their movement. Very strong intermolecular forces contribute to a solid having a definite shape and volume. Furthermore, a solid is not easily compressible and does not flow easily.

Vaporization, Evaporation, and Condensation

States of matter are able to undergo phase transitions. **Vaporization** refers to the transformation of a solid or liquid into a gas. There are two types of vaporization—evaporation and boiling. **Evaporation** is a surface phenomenon and involves the conversion of a liquid into a gas below the boiling temperature at a given pressure. **Evaporation** is also an important component of the water cycle. Boiling occurs below the surface and involves the conversion of liquid into a gas at or above the boiling temperature.

Condensation represents the conversion of a gas into a liquid. It is the reverse of evaporation. Condensation is also most often synonymous with the water cycle. It is a crucial component of distillation.

Phase Transitions

Matter exists in phases and is mostly in the solid, liquid, or gas form. Solid matter has particles packed closely together. Solids are not compressible because they are already so compact that they are actually vibrating due to the significant attractive and repulsive intermolecular forces. Solids have no flow and do not take the shape of their container. Liquids, on the other hand, have flow because particles are not as tightly packed. They take the shape of their container but are not easily compressible because the particles are still fairly close together. Gas particles are different from solids and liquids in that they are very easily compressible. They are so far apart that intermolecular forces are negligible.

Example

Q. Which of the following is a chief difference between evaporation and boiling?

a. Liquids boil only at the surface while they evaporate equally throughout the liquid.

b. Evaporating substances change from gas to liquid while boiling substances change from liquid to gas.

c. Evaporation happens in nature while boiling is a manmade phenomenon.

d. Evaporation can happen below a liquid's boiling point.

Explanation

Answer. D: Evaporation takes place at the surface of a fluid while boiling takes place throughout the fluid. The liquid will boil when it reaches its boiling or vaporization temperature, but evaporation can happen due to a liquid's volatility. Volatile substances often coexist as a liquid and as a gas, depending on the pressure forced on them. The phase change from gas to liquid is condensation, and both evaporation and boiling take place in nature.

Chemical Reactions

Types of Chemical Reactions
Chemical reactions are characterized by a chemical change in which the starting substances, or reactants, differ from the substances formed, or products. Chemical reactions may involve a change in color, the production of gas, the formation of a precipitate, or changes in heat content. The following are the five basic types of chemical reactions:

XX. Synthesis
YY. Decomposition
ZZ. Displacement
AAA.   Double Displacement
BBB.   Combustion

Balancing Chemical Reactions
Chemical reactions are expressed using chemical equations. Chemical equations must be balanced with equivalent numbers of atoms for each type of element on each side of the equation. The reactants are located on the left side of the arrow, while the products are located on the right side of the arrow. Coefficients are the numbers in front of the chemical formulas. Subscripts are the numbers to the lower right of chemical symbols in a formula. To tally atoms, one should multiply the formula's coefficient by the

subscript of each chemical symbol. For example, the chemical equation $2 H_2 + O_2 \rightarrow 2H_2O$ is balanced.

Catalysts

Catalysts are substances that accelerate the speed of a chemical reaction. A catalyst remains unchanged throughout the course of a chemical reaction. Catalysts increase the rate of a chemical reaction by providing an alternate path requiring less activation energy. Activation energy refers to the amount of energy required for the initiation of a chemical reaction. Catalysts can be homogeneous or heterogeneous.

Enzymes

Enzymes are a class of catalysts instrumental in biochemical reactions. Like all catalysts, enzymes increase the rate of a chemical reaction by providing an alternate path requiring less activation energy. Enzymes are proteins and possess an active site, which is the part of the molecule that binds the reacting molecule, or substrate. The "lock and key" analogy is used to describe the substrate key fitting precisely into the active site of the enzyme lock to form an enzyme-substrate complex.

pH, Acids, and Bases

pH refers to the power or potential of hydrogen atoms and is used as a scale for a substance's acidity. The pH scale is a logarithmic scale used to quantify how acidic or basic a substance is. pH is the negative logarithm of the hydrogen ion concentration: pH = -log [H⁺]. A one-unit change in pH correlates with a ten-fold change in hydrogen ion concentration. The pH scale typically ranges from zero to 14, although it is possible to have pHs outside of this range. Pure water has a pH of 7, which is considered neutral. pH values less than 7 are considered acidic, while pH values greater than 7 are considered basic, or alkaline:

Protons, Neutrons, and Electrons

Protons are found in the atomic nucleus and are positively charged particles. The addition or removal of protons from an atom's nucleus creates an entirely different element. **Neutrons** are also found in the atomic nucleus and are neutral particles, meaning they have no net electrical charge. The addition or removal of neutrons from an atom's nucleus does not create a different element but instead creates a lighter or heavier form of that element called an isotope. **Electrons** are found orbiting in the atomic shells around the nucleus and are negatively charged particles. A proton or a neutron has nearly 2,000 times the mass of an electron.

Electrons and Chemical Bonds
Electrons orbit the nucleus in atomic shells, or electron clouds. For example, the first atomic shell can accommodate two electrons, the second atomic shell can hold a maximum of eight electrons, and the third atomic shell can house a maximum of eight electrons.

Chemical bonding typically results in the formation of a new substance, called a compound. Only the electrons in the outermost atomic shell are able to form chemical bonds. These electrons are known as valence electrons, and they are what determines the chemical properties of an atom.

Chemical Bonds Between Atoms
Chemical bonds refer to the manner in which atoms are attached to one another. Atoms may be held together with three fundamental types of chemical bonds—ionic, covalent, or hydrogen.

Ionic Bonding

In an **ionic bond**, an atom loses one or more electrons to another who gains them. The atoms do this so that they can achieve a full outermost shell of electrons, which is the configuration with the lowest amount of energy, and these are typically the strongest types of bonds.

Covalent Bonding

In a **covalent bond**, two or more atoms share one or more electrons. Covalent bonds are the most plentiful type of bond making up the human body. They are typically found in molecules containing carbon. Only six elements typically form covalent bonds: carbon (C), nitrogen (N), phosphorus (P), oxygen (O), sulfur (S), and hydrogen (H).

Hydrogen Bonding

Hydrogen bonds are temporary and weak. They typically occur between two partial, opposite electrical charges. For example, hydrogen bonds form when a hydrogen (H) atom in the vicinity of nitrogen (N), fluorine (F), or oxygen (O) atoms. These partial electrical charges are called dipoles and are caused by the unequal sharing of electrons between covalent bonds. Water is the most prevalent molecule that forms hydrogen bonds.

Example

Q. Most catalysts found in biological systems are which of the following?

    a. Special lipids called cofactors.

    b. Special proteins called enzymes.

    c. Special lipids called enzymes.

    d. Special proteins called cofactors.

Explanation

Answer. B: Biological catalysts are termed *enzymes*, which are proteins with conformations that specifically manipulate reactants into positions which decrease the reaction's activation energy.

Scientific Reasoning

Including Technology and Mathematics in Science Research

Technology is always advancing, and its application is playing an increasingly larger role in science research. Technology increases the accuracy and precision of scientific data, which in many ways is becoming more dependent on the type of technology adopted. Mathematics has been around for centuries and has constantly been called upon in scientific research to help understand and explain the workings of the natural world. It is a crucial part of the scientific

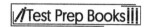

method. Mathematics can help improve and refine the asking of questions or hypotheses in a scientific argument.

Critiquing a Scientific Explanation

A scientific explanation has three crucial components—a claim, evidence, and logical reasoning. A claim makes an assertion or conclusion focusing on the original question or problem. The evidence provides backing for the claim and is usually in the form of scientific data. The scientific data must be appropriate and sufficient. The scientific reasoning connects the claim and evidence and explains why the evidence supports the claim.

Relationships Among Events, Objects, and Processes

Cause and Effect
While it is typical for there to be a single cause and a single effect in a relationship, there are many situations that call for a cause to have many effects, such as exploring the effects of a certain event. In exploring the effects of exercise, for example, the cause is exercise. Effects are stress relief, increased energy, and weight loss.

Unit Size

In understanding relationships between objects
encountered in science, it's important to understand
the scale of them. This is accomplished by
understanding the size of different units of
measurement.

Design of a Scientific Investigation

The scientific method provides the framework for
studying and learning about the world in a scientific
fashion. There is no consensus as to the number of
steps involved in executing the scientific method, but
the following six steps are needed to fulfill the criteria
for correct usage of the scientific method:

CCC.	Ask a question
DDD.	Make observations
EEE.	Create or propose a hypothesis
FFF.	Formulate an experiment
GGG.	Test the hypothesis
HHH.	Accept or reject the hypothesis

Example

Q. A student believes that there is an inverse
relationship between sugar consumption and test
scores. To test this hypothesis, he recruits several
people to eat sugar, wait one hour, and take a short

aptitude test afterwards. The student will compile the participants' sugar intake levels and test scores. How should the student conduct the experiment?

a. One round of testing, where each participant consumes a different level of sugar.

b. Two rounds of testing: The first, where each participant consumes a different level of sugar, and the second, where each participant consumes the same level as they did in Round 1.

c. Two rounds of testing: The first, where each participant consumes the same level of sugar as each other, and the second, where each participant consumes the same level of sugar as each other but at higher levels than in Round 1.

d. One round of testing, where each participant consumes the same level of sugar.

Explanation

Answer. C: To gather accurate data, the student must be able compare a participant's test score from round 1 with their test score from round 2. The differing levels of intellect among the participants means that comparing participants' test scores to those of other participants would be inaccurate.

English and Language Usage

Conventions of Standard English

Standard English Spelling

Below are some guidelines for spelling:

1. Each syllable must have at least one vowel.

2. A short vowel sound indicates only one vowel is needed, such as in *cat* or *red*.

3. Although there are exceptions, remember the saying, "*I* before *e* except after *c* or when sounding as *a* as in *neighbor* or *weigh*."

4. When two vowels are next to each other, the first one makes the sound, and the second one is silent. An example is the word *beam*.

Example

Q. Which of the following uses correct spelling?

 a. Leslie knew that training for the Philadelphia Marathon would take dicsipline and perserverance, but she was up to the challenge.

 b. Leslie knew that training for the Philadelphia Marathon would take discipline and perseverence, but she was up to the challenge.

 c. Leslie knew that training for the Philadelphia Marathon would take disiplin and perservearance, but she was up to the challenge.

 d. Leslie knew that training for the Philadelphia Marathon would take discipline and perseverance, but she was up to the challenge.

Explanation

Answer. D: *Discipline* and *perseverance* are both spelled correctly in Choice *D*. These are both considered commonly misspelled words. One or both words are spelled incorrectly in choices A, B, and C.

Ellipses

An **ellipsis** consists of three dots (. . .) that indicate a word or phrase has been left out of the writing material. Writers will leave words or phrases that are irrelevant to the new text.

Example
Below is an example of an ellipsis being used.

Exercise is good for unexpected reasons. Watkins writes, "Exercise has many benefits such as . . . reducing cancer risk."

Explanation
In the example above, the ellipsis takes the place of the other benefits of exercise that are more expected.

Commas

A **comma** (,) is a punctuation mark that has several different purposes. Sometimes a comma is used to set apart a word or a phrase in a sentence, or sometimes it is used to set off an introductory clause. Here is a list of comma usage:

In a complex sentence, if a subordinate clause comes before the main clause, a comma is placed after the subordinate clause: "After the game was over, we went to the best restaurant in town."

Two commas are used on either side of an interrupting word or phrase: "Our teacher, Mrs. Dowlen, taught us how to use a compass."

An introductory or interrupting phrase at the beginning of a sentence: "While feeding her puppy, Heather realized he also needed water."

A comma should go after an interjection: "Oh yes, I love that movie."

A comma should be used to list two or more items in a sequence: "My favorite foods are lobster, corn, and potatoes."

When expressing a date, commas should go after the month and day, preceding the year. If there is a day of the week, commas should follow that as well, before expressing the date.

Example

Q. Which example shows correct comma usage for dates?

a. The due date for the final paper in the course is Monday, May 16, 2016.
b. The due date for the final paper in the course is Monday, May 16 2016.
c. The due date for the final project in the course is Monday, May, 16, 2016.
d. The due date for the final project in the course is Monday May 16, 2016.

Explanation

Answer. A: It is necessary to put a comma between the date and the year. It is also required to put a comma between the day of the week and the month.

Semicolons

The **semicolon** (;) is a punctuation mark with a couple different uses. Let's look at them below.

> A semicolon separates two independent clauses: "I will walk to school; I will not take the bus."

> The semicolon separates a list of items that already contains a comma: "Last summer we travelled to Austin, Texas; Boise, Idaho; and Little Rock, Arkansas."

Example

Q. Which of the following sentences uses correct punctuation?

    a. Carole is not currently working; her focus is on her children at the moment.
    b. Carole is not currently working and her focus is on her children at the moment.
    c. Carole is not currently working, her focus is on her children at the moment.
    d. Carole is not currently working her focus is on her children at the moment.

Explanation

Answer. A: Choice *A* is correctly punctuated because it uses a semicolon to join two independent clauses that are related in meaning. Each of these clauses could function as an independent sentence.

Colons

Colons (:) have a few different uses listed below.

    III. Colons can be used to introduce a list: "I brought the following drinks: iced tea, lemonade, and water."

    JJJ. Colons can also be used after the greeting in a letter: "Dear Madam:"

    KKK.   Colons are used in the writing of time: "The clock says 12:30 pm."

Example

Q. Which of the following examples uses correct punctuation?

    a. Recommended supplies for the hunting trip include the following: rain gear, large backpack, hiking boots, flashlight, and non-perishable foods.

    b. I left the store, because I forgot my wallet.

    c. As soon as the team checked into the hotel; they met in the lobby for a group photo.

    d. None of the furniture came in on time: so they weren't able to move in to the new apartment.

Explanation

Answer. A: In this example, a colon is correctly used to introduce a series of items.

Hyphens

The **hyphen** is a small dash mark (-) used to link words together. Let's look at a few uses below:

Hyphens are used to create compound adjectives: "free-range eggs."

Some words are built with hyphens, such as "merry-go-round," or "well-being."

Example

Q. Which of the following sentences correctly uses a hyphen?

a. Last-year, many of the players felt unsure of the coach's methods.

b. Some of the furniture she selected seemed a bit over-the-top for the space.

c. Henry is a beagle-mix and is ready for adoption this weekend.

d. Geena works to maintain a good relationship with her ex-husband to the benefit of their children.

Explanation
Answer. D: Choice *D* correctly places a hyphen after the prefix *ex* to join it to the word *husband.* Words that begin with the prefixes *great*, *trans*, *ex*, *all*, and *self*, require a hyphen.

Parentheses

Parentheses () are used in a sentence to offer an aside, a short definition, reference, or an explanation. Let's look at a short example.

Example
"The pie chart of her finances (see below) indicates that her car note is her biggest expense."

Explanation
The words (see below) act as a reference to the pie chart outside of the text and are best put in parentheses.

En-Dash

An en-dash (–) is used to mean "through" by marking a set of dates or a set of numbers, like 1930–1950, or 1–10. It is also used behind affixes.

Example
The affix *circum–* originates from Latin and means *around or surrounding.*

Em-Dash

The em-dash (—) is used to set apart words or a phrase inside of a text. It is longer than a hyphen (-) and an en-dash (–). Using an em-dash within a text sets phrases apart like the parentheses, but unlike the parentheses, draws more attention to the aside.

Example
"Despite rampant coulrophobia—an irrational fear of clowns—Bobo still books more parties and receives higher rates of compensation per show."

Quotation Marks

Let's look at some rules concerning quotation marks:

LLL. Quotation marks are used by authors to create dialogue: Henry replied, "The horses have come back."

MMM.   Quotation marks are used around short stories, titles of poems, titles of songs, essays, and book chapters.

NNN.   Quotation marks are used to emphasize a certain word: The word "permit" is used to indicate authorization.

Example

Q. Which of the following examples correctly uses quotation marks?

    a. "Where the Red Fern Grows" was one of my favorite novels as a child.

    b. Though he is famous for his roles in films like "The Great Gatsby" and "Titanic," Leonardo DiCaprio has never won an Oscar.

    c. Sylvia Plath's poem, "Daddy" will be the subject of this week's group discussion.

    d. "The New York Times" reported that many fans are disappointed in some of the trades made by the Yankees this off-season.

Explanation

Answer. C: Choice *C* is correct because quotation marks should be used for the title of a short work, such as a poem.

Apostrophes

The apostrophe (') has a few different functions we will look at below:

    OOO.   Apostrophes are used to designate a quote within a quote: The professor said, "The word 'circumvent' means to avoid or get around."

PPP.   Apostrophes are used for contractions, such as in "can't" or "won't."

QQQ.   Apostrophes are used to show possession: "Bob's house" or "Veronica's purse."

Example

Q. Which of the following sentences shows correct word usage?

a. It's often been said that work is better then rest.

b. Its often been said that work is better then rest.

c. It's often been said that work is better than rest.

d. Its often been said that work is better than rest.

Explanation

Answer. C: This question focuses on the correct usage of the commonly confused word pairs of *it's/its* and *then/than*. *It's* is a contraction for *it is* or *it has*. *Its* is a possessive pronoun. The word *than* shows comparison between two things. *Then* is an adverb that conveys time.

Types of Sentences

There are four types of sentences in the English language. Let's look at them below:

RRR. **Declarative**: A statement that ends with a period. Example: We are going to the beach this weekend.

SSS. **Imperative**: A command that ends with a period. Example: Clean your room before we go to the beach.

TTT. **Interrogative**: Asks a question. Example: Are we going to my favorite beach?

UUU. **Exclamatory**: A statement that expresses some kind of emotion, usually ending with an exclamation mark. Example: I love going to that beach!

Example

Q. Which of the following is an imperative sentence?

a. Pennsylvania's state flag includes two draft horses and an eagle.

b. Go down to the basement and check the hot water heater for signs of a leak.

c. You must be so excited to have a new baby on the way!

d. How many countries speak Spanish?

Explanation

Answer. B: Choice *B* is an imperative sentence because it issues a command. In addition, it ends with a period, and an imperative sentence must end in a period or exclamation mark.

Knowledge of Language

Nouns

A **noun** is a person, place, thing, or idea. Let's look at the two types of nouns below.

Common Noun

A **common noun** is a word that names general people, places, or things. Examples of common nouns are animals, objects, feelings, actions, qualities, or numbers.

Proper Noun

A **proper noun** is a specific name of a person, place or thing. Examples include names of people, shops, cities, restaurants, churches, banks, or anything with a particular name.

Example

Read the sentence below and then answer the question that follows.

Robert needed to find at least four sources for his final project, so he searched several library databases for reliable academic research.

Which words function as nouns in the preceding sentence?

   a. Robert, sources, project, databases, research
   b. Robert, sources, final, project, databases, academic, research
   c. Robert, sources, project, he, library, databases, research
   d. Sources, project, databases, research

Explanation

Answer. A: Choice *A* includes all of the words functioning as nouns in the sentence.

Pronoun

A **pronoun** is a word used in place of a noun. Here is a list of personal pronouns below:

   VVV.   Personal pronouns: refer to people
   WWW.   First person: we, I, our, mine
   XXX.   Second person: you, yours
   YYY.   Third person: he, them
   ZZZ.   Possessive pronouns: demonstrate ownership (mine, my, his, yours)
   AAAA.   Interrogative pronouns: ask questions (what, which, who, whom, whose)
   BBBB.   Relative pronouns: include the five interrogative pronouns and others that are

relative (whoever, whomever, that, when, where)

CCCC.   Demonstrative pronouns: replace something specific (this, that, those, these)

DDDD.   Reciprocal pronouns: indicate something was done or given in return (each other, one another)

EEEE.   Indefinite pronouns: have a nonspecific status (anybody, whoever, someone, everybody, somebody)

Example

Q. The realtor showed _____ and _____ a house on Wednesday afternoon.

Which of the following pronoun pairs should be used in the blanks above?

a. She, I
b. She, me
c. Me, her
d. Her, me

Explanation

Answer. D: The object pronouns *her* and *me* act as the indirect objects of the sentence. If *me* is in a series of object pronouns, it should come last in the series.

Adjectives

An **adjective** is a word or phrase that describes a noun or pronoun, naming its characteristics. Let's look at a few examples of adjectives below. Adjectives will be underlined.

FFFF.   The girl and her <u>amicable</u> dog went to the park.

GGGG.   Billy's mother went to see a <u>horror</u> movie.

Above, the adjectives describe *what type* of dog and movie. Adjectives describe the size, shape, age color, origin, personality, or type of nouns.

<u>Example</u>
Q. In which of the following sentences does the word *part* function as an adjective?

a. The part Brian was asked to play required many hours of research.

b. She parts ways with the woodsman at the end of the book.

c. The entire team played a part in the success of the project.

d. Ronaldo is part Irish on his mother's side of the family.

Explanation

Answer. D: In Choice *D*, the word *part* functions as an adjective that modifies the word *Irish*.

Possessives

Possessive nouns and pronouns show ownership, such as the word *your*. **Singular nouns** are made possessive with an apostrophe and an *s* (*'s*).

HHHH.   My uncle's new car is silver.
IIII. The dog's bowl is empty.
JJJJ. James's ties are becoming outdated.

Plural nouns ending in *s* are generally made possessive by just adding an apostrophe ('):

KKKK.   The pistachio nuts' saltiness is added during roasting. (The saltiness of pistachio nuts is added during roasting.)
LLLL.   The students' achievement tests are difficult. (The achievement tests of the students are difficult.)

Example

Q. Which of the following sentences shows correct word usage?

    a. Your going to have to put you're jacket over there.

    b. You're going to have to put your jacket over there.

    c. Your going to have to put you're jacket over they're.

    d. You're going to have to put you're jacket over their.

Explanation

Answer. B: Choice *B* correctly uses the contraction for *you are* as the subject of the sentence, and it correctly uses the possessive pronoun *your* to indicate ownership of the jacket. It also correctly uses the adverb *there*, indicating place.

Verbs

The **verb** is the part of speech that describes an action, state of being, or occurrence.

A verb forms the main part of a predicate of a sentence. This means that the verb explains what the noun is doing. A simple example is "Sheila <u>bakes</u> the cake." The verb *bakes* explains what the action of the noun, *Sheila*, is doing.

Example

A student wants to rewrite the following sentence.

Entrepreneurs use their ideas to make money.

Q. The student wants to use the word *money* as a verb, but he isn't sure which word ending to use. What is the appropriate suffix to add to *money* to complete the following sentence?

Entrepreneurs _____ their ideas.

a. –ize
b. –ical
c. –en
d. –ful

Explanation

Answer. A: Only two of these suffixes, *–ize* and *–en*, can be used to form verbs, so *B* and *D* are incorrect. Those choices create adjectives. The suffix *–ize* means "to convert or turn into." The suffix *–en* means "to become." Because this sentence is about converting ideas into money, money + *–ize* or *monetize* is the most appropriate word to complete the sentence, so *C* is incorrect.

Adverbs

Adverbs answer any of the following questions: *How, when, where, why, in what way, how often, how much, in what condition,* and/or *to what degree.*

Example: How good looking is he? He is very handsome.

Here are some examples of adverbs for different situations:

- how: quickly
- when: daily
- where: there
- in what way: easily
- how often: often
- how much: much
- in what condition: badly
- what degree: hardly

Example
Q. The underlined portion of the sentence is an example of which sentence component?

New students should report <u>to the student center</u>.

   a. Dependent clause
   b. Adverbial phrase
   c. Adjective clause
   d. Noun phrase

Explanation
Answer. B: In this case, the phrase functions as an adverb modifying the verb *report*, so *B* is the correct answer.

Prepositions

Prepositions are connecting words that describe relationships. They are placed before a noun or pronoun, forming a phrase that modifies another word in the sentence. **Prepositional phrases** begin with a preposition and end with a noun or pronoun, the **object of the preposition**.

Example
A pristine lake is <u>near the store</u> and <u>behind the bank</u>.

Interjections

Interjections are words used to express emotion. Examples include *wow*, *ouch*, and *hooray*.

<u>Example</u>
<u>Oh no</u>, I am not going.

Conjunctions

Conjunctions are vital words that connect words, phrases, thoughts, and ideas. Conjunctions show relationships between components. There are two types: coordinating and subordinating.

The **coordinating conjunctions** are for, and, nor, but, or, yes, and so. A useful memorization trick is to remember that the first letter of these conjunctions collectively spell the word FABOYS.

The **subordinating conjunctions** connect two unequal parts, one **main** and the other **subordinate**. Example: I must go to the store <u>even though</u> I do not have enough money in the bank.

Example
The underlined words below are examples of conjunctions.

I need to go shopping, <u>but</u> I must be careful to leave enough money in the bank.

She wore a black, red, <u>and</u> white shirt.

Subject-Verb Agreement

The subject of a sentence and its verb must agree. The cornerstone rule of subject-verb agreement is that the subject and verb must agree in number.

MMMM.   Incorrect: The houses is new.
NNNN.   Correct: The houses are new.
OOOO.   Also Correct: The house is new.

Example
Q. Which of the following sentences uses correct subject-verb agreement?
a. There is two constellations that can be seen from the back of the house.
b. At least four of the sheep needs to be sheared before the end of summer.
c. Lots of people were auditioning for the singing competition on Saturday.
d. Everyone in the group have completed the assignment on time.

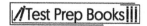

<u>Explanation</u>

Answer. C: The simple subject of this sentence, the word *lots*, is plural. It agrees with the plural verb form *were*.

Formal and Informal Language

Formal language is used in academia or in professional settings. Formal language uses standard English grammar and technical or relevant jargon related to its topic.

Informal language is how one communicates with their peers, family members, or friends. It is not as much concerned with sounding professional, but in communicating in a friendly or casual manner.

Example

Q. A teacher wants to counsel a student about using the word *ain't* in a research paper for a high school English class. What advice should the teacher give?

a. *Ain't* is not in the dictionary, so it isn't a word.
b. Because the student isn't in college yet, *ain't* is an appropriate expression for a high school writer.
c. *Ain't* is incorrect English and should not be part of a serious student's vocabulary because it sounds uneducated.
d. *Ain't* is a colloquial expression, and while it may be appropriate in a conversational setting, it is not standard in academic writing.

Explanation

Answer. D: Colloquial language is that which is used conversationally or informally, in contrast to professional or academic language.

Elements of the Writing Process

The most important parts of the writing process are brainstorming, outlining, writing, referencing sources, and revising. Let's take a better look at them below:

Brainstorming: Before a writer begins their draft, taking a few moments to gather their thoughts, or brainstorming, will make writing easier. Brainstorming also includes jotting down any ideas that come to mind.

Outlining: Outlining a passage means to organize the brainstorming ideas into something cohesive. Writers may outline the introduction, the body paragraphs, and the conclusion. A standard five-paragraph essay outline is below, although essays should always be organized according to the writer's information.

PPPP.	I. Introduction
QQQQ.	II. Topic 1
RRRR.	III. Topic 2
SSSS.	IV. Topic 3
TTTT.	V. Conclusion

Writing: The writing, or drafting, process should follow the outline closely, so the passage doesn't get cluttered.

Referencing sources: Any references to another source should be followed by a citation. Writers should find out which style manual fits their writing best, whether it be APA, MLA, or Chicago style. If using direct quotes, writers should always use quotation marks.

Revising: Read the entire paper and check for any confusing syntax or jumbled ideas. Rewrite where needed. Then, check the paper once more for any grammatical mistakes. This will ensure the essay will be presented at its best.

Example

Q. Which of the following sentences has an error in capitalization?

a. The East Coast has experienced very unpredictable weather this year.

b. My Uncle owns a home in Florida, where he lives in the winter.

c. I am taking English Composition II on campus this fall.

d. There are several nice beaches we can visit on our trip to the Jersey Shore this summer.

Explanation

Answer. B: In Choice *B*, the word *Uncle* should not be capitalized, because it is not functioning as a proper noun. If the word named a specific uncle, such as *Uncle Jerry*, then it would be considered a proper noun and should be capitalized.

Developing a Well-Organized Paragraph

A good *paragraph* should have the following characteristics:

- Be logical with organized sentences

- Have a unified purpose within itself
- Use sentences as building blocks
- Be a distinct section of a piece of writing
- Present a single theme introduced by a topic sentence
- Maintain a consistent flow through subsequent, relevant, well-placed sentences
- Tell a story of its own or have its own purpose, yet connect with what is written before and after
- Enlighten, entertain, and/or inform

Example

Let's examine the following two paragraphs, each an example of a movie review. Read them and form a critique.

Example 1: *Eddie the Eagle* is a movie about a struggling athlete. Eddie was crippled at birth. He had a lot of therapy and he had a dream. Eddie trained himself for the Olympics. He went far away to learn how to ski jump. It was hard for him, but he persevered. He got a coach and kept trying. He qualified for the Olympics. He was the only one from Britain who could jump. When he succeeded, they named him, "Eddie the Eagle."

Example 2: The last movie I saw in the theater was *Eddie the Eagle,* a story of extraordinary perseverance inspired by real life events. Eddie was born in England with a birth defect that he slowly but surely overcame, but not without trial and error (not the least of which was his father's perpetual *dis*couragement). In fact, the old man did everything to get him to give up, but Eddie was dogged beyond anyone in the neighborhood; in fact, maybe beyond anyone in the whole town or even the whole world! Eddie, simply, did not know to quit. As he grew up, so did his dream; a strange one, indeed, for someone so unaccomplished: to compete in the Winter Olympics as a ski jumper (which he knew absolutely nothing about). Eddie didn't just keep on dreaming about it. He actually went to Germany and *worked* at it, facing unbelievable odds, defeats, and put-downs by Dad and the other Men in Charge, aka the Olympic decision-makers. Did that stop him? No way! Eddie got a coach and persevered. Then, when he failed, he persevered some more, again and again. You should be able to open up a dictionary, look at the word "persevere," and see a picture of Eddie the Eagle because, when everybody told him he couldn't, he did. The result? He is forever dubbed, "Eddie the Eagle."

Explanation

Both reviews tell something about the movie *Eddie the Eagle*. Does one motivate the reader to want to see the movie more than the other? The second review uses a more passionate tone and figurative language to better appeal to the audience.

Vocabulary Acquisition

Context Clues

Context clues help readers understand unfamiliar words. Below are the different types of context clues.

UUUU.   A **synonym** is a word that has the same meaning as another word. Example: <u>Large</u> boxes are needed to pack <u>big</u> items.

VVVV.   An **antonym** is a word that has the opposite definition of another word. Example: <u>Large</u> boxes are not needed to pack <u>small</u> items.

WWWW.   **Definitions** are sometimes included within a sentence to define uncommon words. Example: They practiced the <u>rumba</u>, a <u>type of dance</u>, for hours on end.

XXXX.   **Explanations** provide context through elaboration. Example: Large boxes holding items weighing over sixty pounds were stacked in the corner.

YYYY.   **Contrast** in a sentence helps readers to know that the unfamiliar word is set in contrast to a familiar one. Example: These <u>minute</u> creatures were much different than the <u>huge</u> mammals that the zoologist was accustomed to dealing with.

Example

The question is based on the following sentence.

As the tour group approached the bottom of Chichen Itza, the prodigious Mayan pyramid, they became nervous about climbing its distant peak.

Q. Based on the context of the sentence, which of the following words shows the correct meaning of the word *prodigious*?

    a. Very large
    b. Famous
    c. Very old
    d. Fancy

Explanation

Answer. A: The word *prodigious* is defined as very impressive, amazing, or large. In this sentence, the meaning can be drawn from the words *they became nervous about climbing its distant peak*, as this would be an appropriate reaction upon seeing a very large peak that's far in the distance.

Analyzing Word Parts

A word can consist of the following:

- root
- root + suffix
- prefix + root
- prefix + root + suffix

Roots are the basic components of words. A **prefix** is a word, letter, or number that is placed before another. A **suffix** is a letter or group of letters added at the end of a word to form another word.

Example
Q. Glorify, fortify, gentrify, acidify

Based on the preceding words, what is the correct meaning of the suffix –*fy*?
- a. Marked by, given to
- b. Doer, believer
- c. Make, cause, cause to have
- d. Process, state, rank

Explanation
Answer. C: The suffix -*fy* means to make, cause, or cause to have. Choices *A, B*, and *D* are incorrect because they show meanings of other suffixes. Choice *A* shows the meaning of the suffix -*ous*. Choice *B*

shows the meaning of the suffix *–ist*, and Choice *D* shows the meaning of the suffix *-age*.

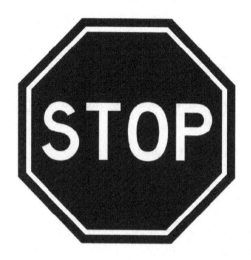

FREE Test Taking Tips DVD Offer

To help us better serve you, we have developed a Test Taking Tips DVD that we would like to give you for FREE. **This DVD covers world-class test taking tips that you can use to be even more successful when you are taking your test.**

145

All that we ask is that you email us your feedback about your study guide. Please let us know what you thought about it – whether that is good, bad or indifferent.

To get your **FREE Test Taking Tips DVD**, email freedvd@studyguideteam.com with "FREE DVD" in the subject line and the following information in the body of the email:

> a. The title of your study guide.

> b. Your product rating on a scale of 1-5, with 5 being the highest rating.

> c. Your feedback about the study guide. What did you think of it?

> d. Your full name and shipping address to send your free DVD.

If you have any questions or concerns, please don't hesitate to contact us at freedvd@studyguideteam.com.

Thanks again!